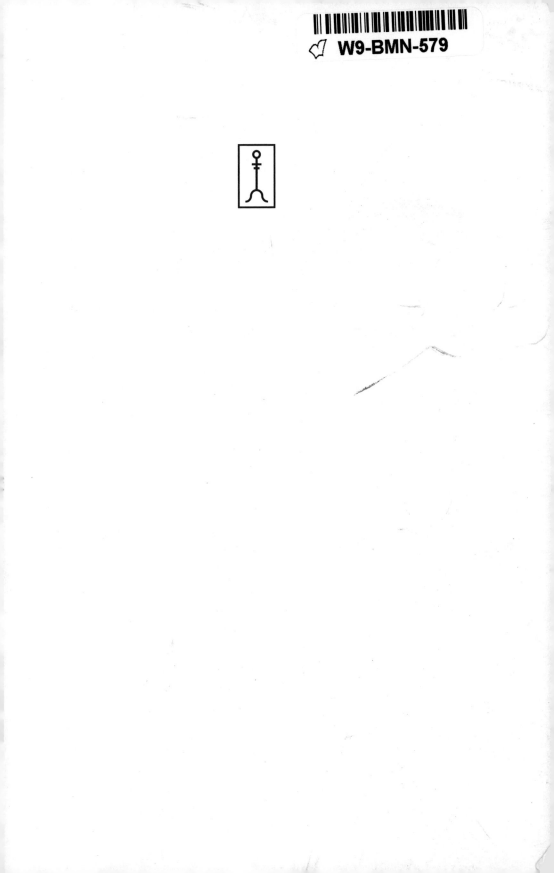

THE
TESTOSTERONE
ADVANTAGE
PLAN™

BY **LOU SCHULER**

WITH **Jeff Volek**, R.D., Ph.D., **Michael Mejia**, AND **Adam Campbell**

A Fireside Book

Published by Simon & Schuster

New York   London   Toronto   Sydney   Singapore

FIRESIDE
Rockefeller Center
1230 Avenue of the Americas
New York, NY 10020

First Fireside Edition 2003

Published by arrangement with Rodale Inc.

FIRESIDE and colophon are registered trademarks of Simon & Schuster, Inc.

For information about special discounts for bulk purchases,
please contact Simon & Schuster Special Sales:
1-800-456-6798 or business@simonandschuster.com

Manufactured in the United States of America

10 9 8 7 6 5 4 3 2

The Library of Congress has cataloged the Rodale edition as follows:

Schuler, Lou.
The Testosterone Advantage Plan / by Lou Schuler ;
with Jeff Volek, Michael Mejia, and Adam Campbell.
p.   cm.
Includes index.
1. Men—Health and hygiene. 2. Men—Nutrition. 3. Physical fitness for men.
4. Testosterone—Physiological effect. I. Title.
RA777.8 .S38 2002
613.7'0449—dc21
2001005549

ISBN 0-7432-3791-9

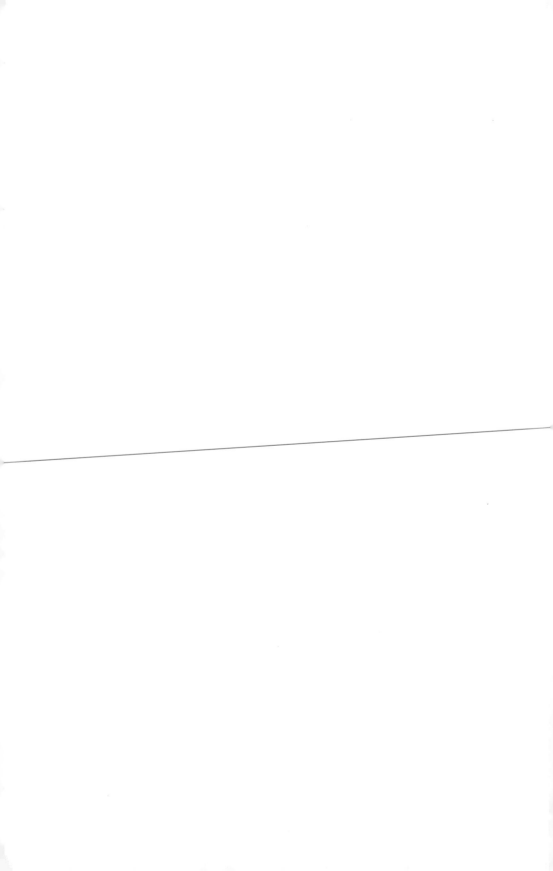

THE TESTOSTERONE ADVANTAGE PLAN™

STAFF

EXECUTIVE EDITOR
Steve Salerno

ASSOCIATE EDITOR
Kathryn C. LeSage

SENIOR DEVELOPMENT EDITOR
Leah Flickinger

ART DIRECTOR
Charles Beasley

COVER AND INTERIOR DESIGNER
Susan P. Eugster

EXERCISE PHOTOGRAPHER
Mitch Mandel

RESEARCH EDITOR
Deborah Pedron

SENIOR RESEARCHER
Deanna Portz

EDITORIAL RESEARCHERS
Christina Bilheimer, Lori Davis, Lynn Goldstein,
Jan McLeod, Elizabeth Price, Bernadette Sukley

LAYOUT DESIGNER
Bethany Bodder

PRODUCT SPECIALIST
Brenda Miller

RODALE *MEN'S HEALTH* BOOKS

VICE PRESIDENT, WORLDWIDE PUBLISHER
Edward J. Fones

MARKETING DIRECTOR
Bob Keppel

ASSOCIATE CUSTOMER MARKETING MANAGER
Matt Neumaier

CONTENT ASSEMBLY MANAGER
Robert V. Anderson Jr.

OFFICE MANAGER
Alice Debus

ASSISTANT OFFICE MANAGER
Marianne Moor

ADMINISTRATIVE ASSISTANT
Pamela Brinar

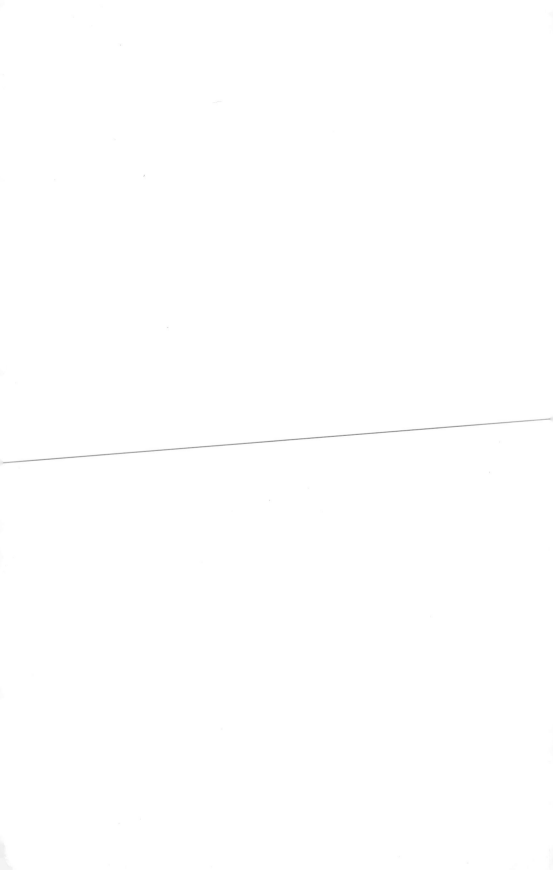

*This book is dedicated to men,
and our eternal struggle
to reach our full potential*

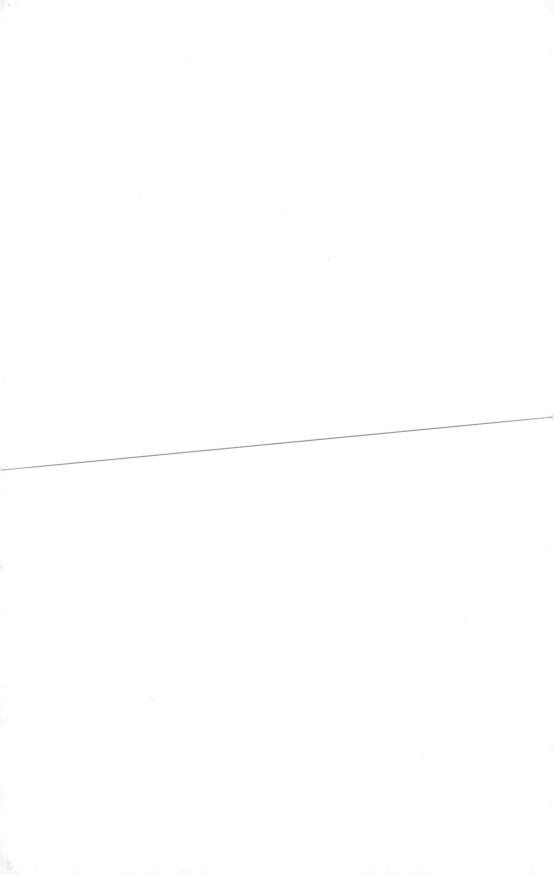

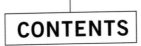

CONTENTS

ACKNOWLEDGMENTS *xiii*

INTRODUCTION *xv*

PART ONE

Chapter 1: **Our Burgers, Ourselves** *3*

Chapter 2: **Why Almost Everything You Know about Fitness Is Probably Dead Wrong** *21*

Chapter 3: **The Cardio Conundrum** *31*

Chapter 4: **Testosterone: A Man's Key to Getting and Staying Fit** *45*

PART TWO

Chapter 5: **The *Men's Health* T** *57*

Chapter 6: **The Meat/Muscle Connection** *61*

Chapter 7: **The Manly Fats** *77*

Chapter 8: **Carbohydrate Revisited** *88*

Chapter 9: **Putting Together the Food Plan** *94*

Chapter 10: **When You Eat, and Why It Matters** *105*

Chapter 11: **The 1-Week Meal Planner** *114*

PART THREE

Chapter 12: **Introduction to the Testosterone Advantage Workout** *155*

Chapter 13: **Getting Ready to Lift** *166*

Chapter 14: **The Testosterone Advantage Workout: Phase 1** *198*

Chapter 15: **The Testosterone Advantage Workout: Phase 2** *226*

Chapter 16: **The Testosterone Advantage Workout: Phase 3** *256*

Chapter 17: **Life at the Top** *285*

ABOUT THE AUTHORS *295*

INDEX *297*

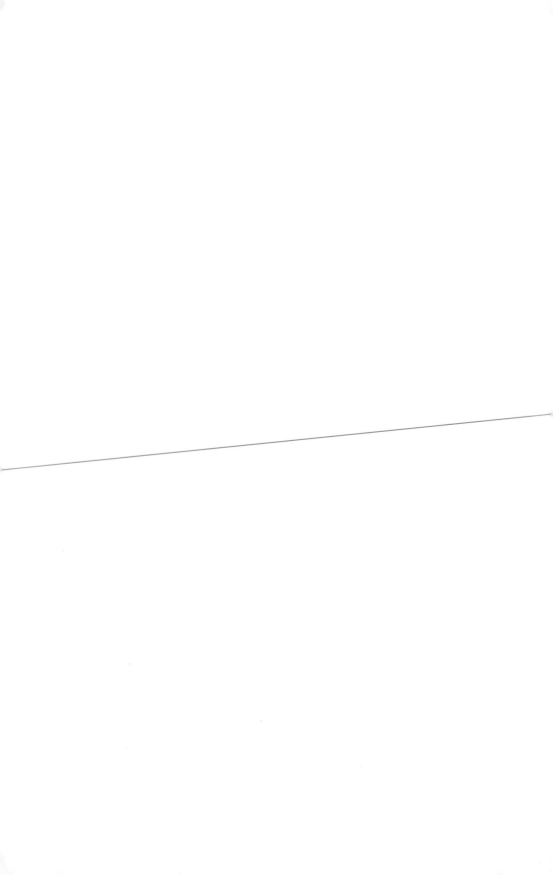

ACKNOWLEDGMENTS

As you can tell by the four names on the cover, *The Testosterone Advantage Plan* was a team effort. Perhaps the most important player is one who's not on the cover. Steve Salerno, executive editor of *Men's Health* Books, had been on the job one week when he sat down with me and Adam Campbell, C.S.C.S., our assistant fitness editor at *Men's Health* magazine, to come up with book ideas.

Steve, Adam, and I had all been reading about higher-fat diets, and we were excited about the theory that guys might be able to lose more weight by adding fat to their diets, rather than eliminating it. I mentioned the benefit of boosting testosterone, and Adam and I talked about how strength training is a better fat-loss tool than aerobic exercise.

From that brief meeting in July 2000, thanks to Steve's relentless and enthusiastic advocacy, a book was born.

I approached Jeff Volek, R.D., Ph.D., C.S.C.S., to whom I'd introduced myself a few weeks earlier at the National Strength and Conditioning Association annual conference, and asked if he could design a diet that would boost testosterone; produce either fat loss or muscle gain, depending on the reader's goals; offer multiple health benefits; and be easy to remember and follow. Jeff, an assistant research professor at the University of Connecticut in Storrs, proved equal to the task, laying the groundwork for the Testosterone Advantage Plan diet in a matter of weeks.

At the same time, I asked *Men's Health* exercise advisor Michael Mejia, C.S.C.S., to provide a workout that would work for both beginning and advanced lifters. Mike and I have worked together for 5 years on various projects for the magazine and menshealth.com, and he has never failed to come through with innovative and effective workouts.

We recruited our co-workers to try out the diet and workouts so we could see whether they really delivered the promised benefit: more muscle with less fat. If the plan hadn't worked, you wouldn't be reading this book right now. The 16 guys who signed on for the 9-week pilot program became walking billboards for the Testosterone Advantage Plan and convinced all of us we were on to something that would benefit a lot of guys frustrated by ineffective diet-and-workout programs.

The job of cobbling together the work of multiple authors fell to associate editor Kathryn C. LeSage and research editor Deborah Pedron. Assembling and organizing the 3-foot stack of research studies backing the claims we make in this book could've kept a lesser researcher busy for a year, but Deb pulled it together in just 3 months.

The final person whose efforts made this book possible is my wife, Kimberly Heinrichs. For 10 months, Kimberly shouldered my parental duties along with her own so that I could write this book in the mornings before work and on weekends. On top of that, she pursued her own freelance writing in the evenings, after the kids and I had gone to bed. This would have been difficult enough, but those 10 months were the most traumatic of her life. In August 2000, she broke her leg in three places—just 10 days before our third child was born. She spent the following 6 weeks in a wheelchair and the ensuing 8 months trying to regain her strength and humor. Whenever I start to feel like Superman for pulling this book together without missing a deadline at the magazine, I have to remind myself that Kimberly was the true superhero.

—L.S.

INTRODUCTION

I've been a true believer in strenuous workouts for as long as I can remember. To me, the passion was always tied up in how I looked. I hated being a weird, skinny kid with glasses. Then I discovered weights. Once I started lifting, I was still weird and had glasses, but I didn't have to be so skinny anymore.

You see, I had an idea, from a very early age, that there was an ideal male shape: wide shoulders, narrow waist, thick chest, muscular arms and legs. I admired the athletes who looked that way—wrestlers, gymnasts, sprinters, some football players. If I couldn't physically do the things they could do, at least I could look like them. I could have that shape.

It's the same shape the ancient Greeks and Romans idealized. Wealthy Romans had their facial likenesses sculpted onto the statues of young, muscular athletes so people would remember them as having attained ideal bodily proportions—even though they didn't actually look like that.

And it wasn't just human representations: The Greeks and Romans—and most artists who followed—chose this shape for their depictions of the deities they worshipped. If this is the ideal shape for man, they reasoned, it must be the very embodiment of the gods themselves.

It's taken a long time for us to get back to the simple intuitive aware-ness of the Greeks and Romans, but once again today, the body men want is the one our forebears admired. The one I grew up wanting to attain. The one women say they most appreciate. I believe that somewhere in our psyches is embedded this image of what an adult human male should look like—a kind of species memory, or maybe a gender one, that wells up in us every so often to remind us what we're supposed to aspire to.

That's why I take issue with the exercise-and-nutrition establishment for pushing exercise that doesn't give us this shape, for touting diets that prevent us from getting or keeping this shape. Together, the self-ap-pointed gurus of diet and exercise claim a world of health benefits would accrue to us *if only we did the things that won't give us this shape.*

And so if you want to slim down, they almost certainly give you a diet-and-exercise program guaranteeing that you'll also lose muscle, slow your metabolism, and lower your testosterone.

On the other hand, if you want to gain solid, muscular weight, you're treated like a freak—given no place to turn but the supplement-ped-dling, circus-sideshow world of bodybuilding.

And if you're generally satisfied with your weight but just want to look more like the guys on the cover of, say, *Men's Health*, you're given advice that makes it nearly impossible to reach that goal.

And for what purpose? Are the establishment's diets healthier? No. The population is fatter than any in several American generations—fully 61 percent of us are fat. With each passing week, more and more of the establishment's sacred nutritional cows are revealed as myth.

Well then, are the establishment's exercise programs healthier? Again, no. New research tells us that strenuous exercise needn't be aerobic to prolong life and prevent disease. Besides which, many of the most pop-ular forms of aerobic exercise have their own health pitfalls.

So what are we trying to accomplish with this book? First of all, we're telling you man-to-man that your instincts are on target: The reason you want to look a certain way is that you're supposed to look that way. It's the natural shape of a strong, fit, healthy male, attained through the ex-ercise-and-diet program in this book. A shape you can maintain for life, if you go about it seriously, consistently, and correctly.

Lifetime maintenance isn't easy, by the way. We don't want to get technical yet, but your metabolism declines with age—2 or 3 percent per decade. This attrition is linked directly to lost muscle mass. One of the primary purposes of this book is to show you how to keep that particular physique-eating wolf away from your door as long as possible.

Are there other paths to the same destination? Perhaps. Ours is just the straightest one we know of. Equally important, our talk is straight too. What we'll offer you is an achievable goal, based on a program you can actually follow to get realistic results. It's not a program built upon hype or junk science; it's not a program in which we hook you with a bunch of gee-wow photos that depend on trick lighting or skillful retouching. As you'll see in the before-and-after stories of the men in our own pilot program, these are real guys, just like you, not one of whom ended up looking like Mr. Olympia. First of all, you're not going to get to Mr. Olympia without injecting foreign substances into your body. And you're not going to get there in 9 weeks, no matter what. (You already knew that, didn't you? You could take every steroid known to man and it would still take you many years of hard training to build that kind of bulk.)

But we have a feeling that if you're honest with yourself, a career in bodybuilding has never been an option or even an ambition. You just want to be the best *you* can be. So this we promise: We're going to give you a helluva head start on a new life. With our program as your guide, you'll never be ashamed to be on the skins side when playing against the shirts. You'll get your share of glances on the beach. Oh, and you'll feel much better than you have in ages.

We're giving you a chance to become what you most admire. We're giving you a program that promotes health, strength, longevity, self-confidence, dynamic energy, and hope for the future.

We're giving you back your manhood.

LOU SCHULER
FITNESS DIRECTOR, *MEN'S HEALTH* MAGAZINE

THE
TESTOSTERONE ADVANTAGE
PLAN™

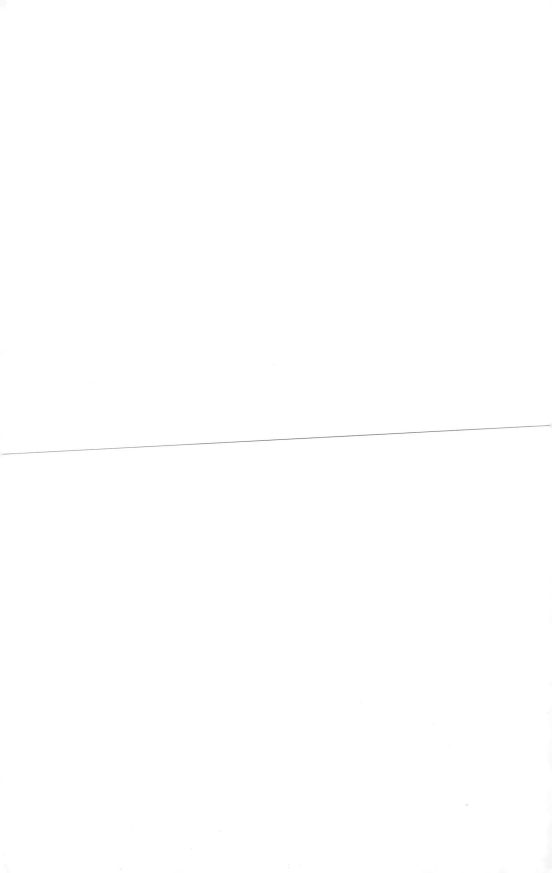

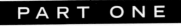

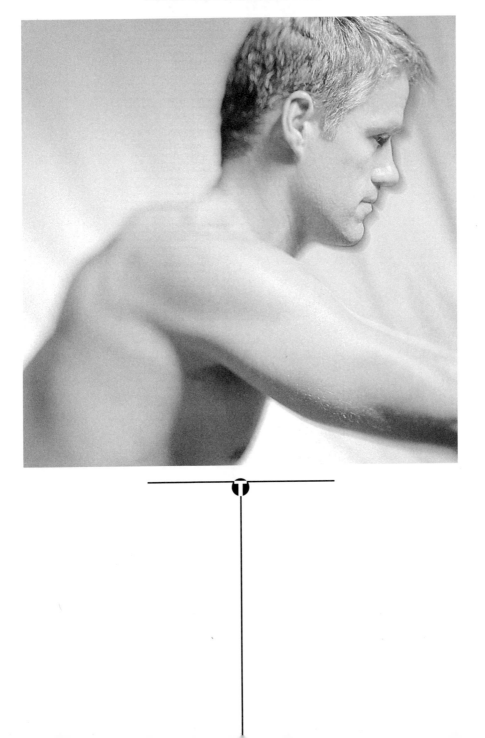

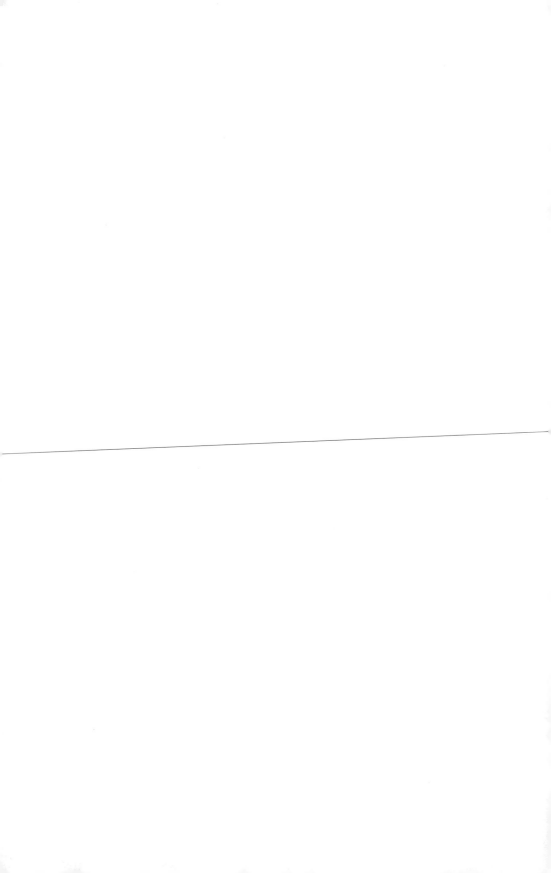

Our Burgers, Ourselves

Are you a man who's interested in looking his best? *Being* his best? Staying physically and physiologically at the top of his game?

We feel for you. We really do.

That's because you've been overlooked. And you've been misled. For 20 years, the fitness and weight-loss industries have had little to offer you. For 20 years, you've been overfed but undernourished. Overworked but underexercised. Overanalyzed but still misunderstood.

Along the way, well-meaning people—often with impressive credentials—have tried to help you. They began by steering you away from the foods you enjoy. When you didn't take an immediate liking to the foods they wanted you to eat instead, other friendly folks in the packaged-food business stepped up with better-tasting versions. When the more palatable food made you fat, yet another group of sincere individuals chimed in to show you a type of exercise that helped you lose some of the fat—but also caused your body to lose a lot of its muscle and your joints to cry out in protest.

At the end of it all, not only are you still out of shape but now you have weak, arthritic knees.

Why? Because all those wonderful diets and fitness programs you were given *don't work*.

Not for you. Not for most men.

You're going to be exposed to a lot of eyebrow-raising notions in this book. We'll tell you that the Food Guide Pyramid doesn't work for us men. A low-fat, high-carbohydrate diet doesn't work for us. (Except, maybe, for the marathoners among us. For the rest of the male population, a low-calorie diet consisting mostly of carbs is a metabolic and physiological disaster waiting to happen.) Most forms of aerobic exercise don't work for us. For that matter, even weight lifting, as you were traditionally taught it—"Grab X number of pounds, lift 10 times, do three sets, repeat"—doesn't work. Not the way it's supposed to.

On what do we base such bold assertions? For starters, decades after the American Heart Association and other leading voices began singing the praises of "low fat" and "exercise," the average guy is more out of shape than his 1960s predecessor. Between 1960 and 1994, the percentage of obese men leaped from 10.4 to 19.9 percent of the total U.S. male population, according to the National Center for Health Statistics.

Sounds pretty bad? Some estimates are worse. Indeed, the latest government statistics tell us that more than half of all Americans are now overweight.

Frankly, we're angry about all this. We're angry with the nutrition establishment, which bullied us into eating less fat, less protein, and much, much more carbohydrate. This much-ballyhooed dietary template has made us fatter than ever before, slowing our metabolisms and screwing with our hormones—specifically, our testosterone.

We're angry with the food industry, which has co-opted the low-fat paradigm and drained whatever virtue it may have contained, replacing fat with sugar and giving us foods we can't stop eating, despite the fact that they never fill us up.

And we're angry with the exercise movement, which decided early on that "fitness" meant "aerobic exercise" and pushed a gullible public into pursuing workout routines that were fine for keeping skinny people skinny but did surprisingly little for the emerging over-weight majority.

None of this had to happen. There's a better way to eat and a better way to exercise.

We're going to present a new paradigm. We're going to present a diet that's based on the healthiest nutritional model in the world, a diet that will allow you to eat less but feel as if you've eaten more, a diet that will increase your metabolism and boost your testosterone. We're going to show you a workout program that will build muscle, further increase your metabolism, and introduce you to the lean, vital man you want to be.

INFLATIONARY TRENDS

We live a lifestyle that's almost designed to make us fat, in a world that's determined to help things along in any way possible. Increasing numbers of us sit in front of computers all day, then go home and sit in front of TVs till bedtime. The Sporting Goods Manufacturers Association tells us that just 20.5 percent of Americans exercised three or more times a week in 1999. Meanwhile, we go out for dinner and manage to pack away 1,000 or more calories before the main course arrives. (Ever share one of those deep-fried onion-wedge appetizers with a buddy or a girlfriend? With the dipping sauce, that's more than 1,000 calories right there. For each of you. There's a difference between "eating more fat" and "eating humongous quantities of crap." All this will become clearer as we move along.) We're drowning in "value meals," offers of two pepperoni pizzas for the price of one, and other incentives to stuff ourselves to the point of self-loathing.

But that alone isn't the problem—or at least, it's not the sole problem. Because guess what? "Eating right" isn't the answer, either. Not the way you were taught to do it, growing up.

At this point we'd like to lay out for you four simple, straightforward truths that will occupy us for the rest of this book.

(continued on page 9)

Why We Overeat

In 2000, the U.S. Centers for Disease Control and Prevention declared that 61 percent of American adults are officially overweight. The first time the government calculated the fat of the land, between 1960 and 1962, a mere 43.5 percent of the population was overweight.

Back then, you almost had to try to be fat. You had to seek out the fattiest foods, like the fancy cream pastries most of the population couldn't afford, except on special occasions. You had to avoid exercise, usually by getting promoted from your manual-labor job into a position that involved a minimum of exertion and a maximum of prestige. Corpulence itself was a status symbol; it meant you had made it in life.

Today, of course, we know that corpulence means something quite different. In fact, it may well mean a quicker exit *out* of life.

Nowadays you have to try to be lean. The issue isn't money so much as time. Sure, it costs less than five bucks to get a 1,970-calorie lunch at Burger King consisting of a Double Whopper with Cheese, a large order of fries, and a large Coke. But it doesn't cost a whole lot more to have a roasted chicken breast, a mixed-green salad with olive oil–based dressing, and a whole wheat roll—a 429-calorie meal with the highest-quality sources of protein, fat, and carbohydrate. Problem is, shopping for, cooking, and eating the good meal takes 2 hours. You don't even have to get out of your car to get the 1,970 fast-food calories. Five minutes in a drive-thru line, another 5 minutes to wolf it down, and you're done, give or take a belch or two.

And that's not even factoring in physical activity—or the lack of same. We've built our world around cars and elevators. We maintain our lawns with riding mowers and leaf blowers. Technological and mechanical advances have taken away even the simplest everyday exertion. We keep files on computer drives instead of in creaky file cabinets that require us to get up out of our ergonomically designed office chairs, walk across the hall, and give a good hard yank on a handle. Electric screwdrivers and nail guns take the physical effort out of household repairs, just as microwaves and electric can openers shave a few calories off the price of food preparation.

You've heard all of this before, and there's not a lot you can do about it. You're not going to throw out your computer or microwave. You're not going to live your life without ever eating fast food. And we aren't going to ask you to. But we will ask you to consider this:

We're Sweetening Ourselves to Death

The U.S. Department of Agriculture says the average American ate 3,800 calories a day in 1994—up from 3,300 calories in 1970. That's 500 more calories per day. If you added that many calories to your diet starting today and didn't compensate with exercise, you'd gain a pound a week. More telling is that the consumption of caloric sweeteners—high-fructose corn syrup and other sugars—increased by about 32 pounds per person per year between 1970 and 1997.

We eat about 20 teaspoons of sugar a day, according to the USDA. At 16 calories per teaspoon, that's 320 calories a day, and 146,000 calories in a year. Add 320 calories to your diet today without additional activity, and within a year you'll gain 33 pounds of fat.

Once You're Fat, It's Easier to Get Fatter

The bigger your waist, the lower your levels of testosterone and the higher your levels of the hormone insulin and the protein leptin, according to a 2001 study in the *International Journal of Obesity*. Appetite is complex and not fully understood, but we do know that insulin and leptin help control it. For example, if you inject insulin into the brain of a rat, it eats less. A rat shot up with leptin has the same response: It eats less. (Needless to say, by the time this is all said and done, you have some really pissed-off rats.)

So theoretically, higher insulin and leptin levels should mean lower appetite and thus a slower fork. But in humans, something happens that throws this off. For example, you could make a good argument that high-sugar diets disrupt the normal appetite-suppressing role of insulin. The sugar creates a spike in blood glucose, and that in turn creates a spike in insulin to clear the glucose out of the blood.

(continued)

Once the glucose is cleared out, hunger kicks in, and you want to eat again.

As for leptin, it's possible that the same process occurs, or that humans are just naturally resistant to high leptin levels. Your body spikes up the levels to suppress your appetite, but then something happens and the leptin either has no effect or the opposite of the intended effect.

Whatever causes these phenomena, the result is a double whammy for men. Your appetite isn't suppressed, so you eat more and you get fatter. And when you get fatter, you decrease testosterone, thus creating a second problem by cutting off one of your body's most potent fat-fighting weapons. It's like hitting Superman with kryptonite. You're left with sugar being rapidly stored around your midsection in the form of fat, and your fat-fighting superhero is rendered helpless.

But What about Genetics?

We admit that we've greatly simplified the weight-control equation. Lots more is involved, principally including genetics, which has a very strong effect on fat storage in the chest and abdomen.

Another wild card is brain chemistry. A 2001 study in *The Lancet* found a connection between obesity and faulty brain wiring that minimizes the brain's reaction to a hormone called dopamine. You know who else has been found to have fewer dopamine receptors? Drug addicts and people with attention-deficit disorder (ADD). A drug addict takes cocaine or methamphetamine to feel normal. A guy with ADD takes Ritalin. And an obese person eats.

The researchers found that the dopamine-obesity relationship is linear. That is, the fatter you are, the fewer dopamine receptors your brain has. Dopamine receptors could shut down as you get fatter, eat more, and generate more dopamine. This would be your brain's way of saying, "Hey, I've got enough dopamine up here." But in response, you'd just keep eating, creating more dopamine as reinforcements in the search for the ever-fewer receptors that would tell you to stop eating.

However, the researchers concede that it's possible the cause and effect could go in the other direction: It could be that the people who are destined to be fattest start life with the fewest dopamine receptors.

Either way, a lack of receptors is damned good news for the trailer-park crystal meth industry. And it's bad news for overweight guys trying to slim down.

FACT ONE: Low-fat diets lower testosterone, making it harder to build muscle and easier to store fat.

FACT TWO: Aerobic exercise programs make it still harder to build muscle. Not only is there no muscle-building stimulus, there are actually muscle-*eroding* physiological shifts associated with serious endurance exercise. And it's hard on the joints to boot.

FACT THREE: Less muscle means a slower metabolism—which means still more fat down the road.

FACT FOUR: Since weight training can enhance the structural integrity of joints and connective tissues—rather than wear them down—it stands to reason that it should be the first exercise choice for men.

So what happened here? How did we get so far removed from the kind of diet-and-exercise regimen that really works for men?

Let's go back to the Food Guide Pyramid for a moment. In 1980, the U.S. government formalized a series of Dietary Guidelines that were themselves an outgrowth of the "four food groups" model that began to take hold during the 1950s. The Food Guide Pyramid was created in 1992 and added to the Dietary Guidelines in 1995 as a teaching tool to illustrate the number of servings that you should eat

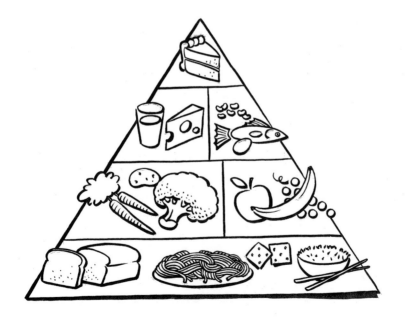

U.S. Department of Agriculture and
U.S. Department of Health and Human Services

from each food group. Today, the main USDA mantra is "Let the pyramid guide your food choices." Basically, it emphasizes large amounts of carbohydrate (the so-called healthy base of the pyramid), somewhat smaller amounts of fruits and vegetables, even smaller amounts of protein, and very, very small amounts of fat. It bears noting that the final shaping and composition of the pyramid was not exactly a scientifically pristine process, as many groups (including the meat and dairy industries) lobbied the USDA as well as the Department of Health and Human Services to protect their interests in the matter.

Nonetheless, even if we take the Food Guide Pyramid at face value, there are so many errors and inconsistencies as to make it functionally worthless as a tool for governing our dietary choices.

For starters, while the pyramid sets forth a fairly straightforward account of the relative amounts we should be eating from the major food groups, it makes no distinctions among the legitimate subcategories that exist within each group. For instance, in the pyramid, grains are grains, whether you're talking about a hearty bowl of old-fashioned oatmeal or a nutritionally worthless slice of white bread—and despite the huge differences in the nutritional and metabolic values of whole grain and refined flour (vitamin enrichment aside).

In the same way, though the Food Guide Pyramid does not specifically mention proteins by name, it lumps most types of protein-based foods in the same group, even though nutritionists say animal proteins (like the burgers we love) are a more complete form of protein than vegetable proteins in their ability to provide B vitamins and essential amino acids. Neither does the pyramid take into account the fact that there's a world of difference between a helping of salmon, which is rich in heart-healthy omega-3 oils, and a helping of bologna, which is rich in not very much. Just as bad—maybe even worse, for our purposes—all fats are imprisoned together in a tiny cell at the top (and remember, in the pyramid, the higher you go, the less desirable a food supposedly is). As a final insult, the sweets are also thrown right in there with the fats.

Thus, in the maddeningly simplistic hierarchy of government-sponsored eating, healthy fats like olive and fish oils are equal partners with dough-nuts and DingDongs.

Now and then, you'll hear the pyramid's defenders point to the de-clining death rate from heart disease as evidence that the pyramid is paying dividends. To this we reply: Nonsense. To credit the pyramid alone with the drop in cardiac mortality is to ignore the major advances in cardiac surgery and drug therapy over the past few decades. That's an omission bordering on fraud. And ask yourself this: If the Food Guide Pyramid were really making Americans healthier, wouldn't it also be making them thinner? In other words, if the pyramid is responsible for declining cardiac death rates, that must mean an awful lot of people are using it to plan their meals. But if that's the case—and if the pyramid ac-tually does what it says it does—then *why the hell is America so fat*? No less a bastion of conventional thought than the Harvard School of Public Health itself conceded, in a study reported in the November 2000 *American Journal of Clinical Nutrition*, that the pyramid was "only weakly associated" with a lessened risk of major diseases like heart attack and cancer.

Others claim that the real problem here is compliance, that when you come right down to it, not that many people follow the pyramid's rec-ommendations after all. Fair enough—but such a contention, if true, completely undercuts any claims about the pyramid's positive effects on American health. How could the pyramid be uplifting the face of heart health if nobody really pays attention to it?

So we don't buy the noncompliance alibi for a minute. And if you're married, you don't either. You know from experience that your wife is constantly trying to get you to eat "better," to attempt to follow the nu-trition establishment's guidelines.

To us, this prompts the core issue in this entire debate: whether any-body—particularly an active man—*should* try to eat like that as a way of life.

We're not lone voices in the wilderness, by the way. The American Heart Association, the Harvard School of Public Health, and the Physicians Committee for Responsible Medicine, to name just three, have advocated rethinking the pyramid, to some degree, with a goal toward less simplicity and more realism.

We, on the other hand, would rather see the pyramid junked than refined. Since we know it doesn't work, rejiggering it will only leave people more confused than ever. In its place, we'd like to suggest the *Men's Health* T. Our T, as you may have guessed, stands for testosterone. That's because our diet increases your testosterone by increasing your intake of healthy fat. For the simple fact is: Today's ultra low fat diets are detrimental to us as men.

See, dietary fats don't spend all their time clogging your arteries. Fat cells are a major energy source for vital organs, your heart included. They're the principal carriers and bodily repositories of the all-important fat-soluble vitamins A, D, E, and K, which are stored in fatty tissues and the liver until needed.

But more to the point of this book, in men, they also play a key role in triggering testosterone production. For that reason, we think your diet should include at least 30 percent fat, and perhaps as much as 40 percent.

Of course, if you've been paying attention the past few dozen years, you've heard that 30 percent fat is the maximum a health-conscious person should eat and that we'd all be better off with less than 20 percent. We hope to convince you that such a diet is a nutritional and metabolic disaster for men. And we want you to at least give our higher-fat diet a try. Even without our muscle-building, testosterone-boosting workout plan, the diet should leave you looking lean but never feeling hungry—a hell of a combination in these overinflated times.

You'll get the best results, however, when you combine the diet with the workout plan: Each works fine on its own, but the two create a beautiful synergy in tandem. We learned this from the 16 men who completed our 9-week pilot program. You'll meet some of them throughout the book, in the "Before & After" profiles.

First, however, we'd like you to join us in a little visualization exercise.

(continued on page 16)

Our Pilot Program

We've been pretty cocky about the Testosterone Advantage Plan from the outset. After all, the latest medical literature is clearly on our side. Still, we got tired of reading about other people's tests. So we decided it wouldn't be a bad idea to put some guys on a plan of our own design, to see if we could produce the sorts of results the studies led us to expect.

On a snowy night in early January 2001, we convened 30 volunteers who'd taken us up on the invitation to be our pilot program. We'd picked January because we wanted men who'd be highly motivated—the same type of men who would buy this book. At that time of year, we knew, we'd find guys who were pretty disgusted with themselves after 2 solid months of pigging out.

To qualify for the program, our volunteers had to agree to a few rules. First and foremost, they had to follow the program to a T, as it were—no deviations. Second, they had to perform strength tests at the beginning and end of the 9-week program. Third, they had to report their weight each week so we could track their progress.

We lost some of our volunteers right off the bat, and for reasons besides the dreaded before-and-after photos to which participants also had to agree.

One guy's doctor advised that he abstain from the program. (Apparently, this practitioner thought that his patient would not benefit from losing 25 pounds and exercising regularly—which just goes to show the knee-jerk defensiveness you often encounter when you put something different in front of the medical establishment.) Four guys deemed the plan's grocery-shopping and meal-making elements too complicated. Three guys said they traveled too much to follow the plan with the degree of loyalty we expected. And so on.

When the dust settled, we ended up with 16 committed participants.

Thus began the process of individualizing meal plans for our guys, based upon their respective body-composition goals. This entailed about 6 days in front of the computer, determining the right amounts of protein, fat, and carbohydrate for each guy, and then, in turn, spreading out those amounts over five reasonably appetizing, user-friendly meals per day. Most of the sample meal plans you'll find in this book are byproducts of what we learned in those early calculations.

Then we gave each guy his meal plan and his personal exercise program. And we turned them all loose.

(continued)

Every Monday, they reported the latest good news from the scale or the weight room. Most of them had very few quibbles as the program moved along. For the most part, they were eating food they liked, losing weight, and having fun.

The 9-week results were impressive. Among the participants who had hoped to lose flab, the average drop was 18 pounds; the heaviest guy shed 28 pounds. Those numbers were right in line with our projections. Plus, overall, our guys posted impressive strength gains, and they reported having more energy—not to mention increased sex drives. (Okay, we'll mention it.)

As for those before-and-afters . . . we wanted them to be real pictures of real guys, just like you. We wanted to show what was achievable for a regular guy in a short 9 weeks. We wanted to give you a hint at how much better the results could be for you personally if you stick with the program longer.

So we didn't use trick lighting. And our guys didn't tan, shave their chests, or get new haircuts. Well, that's not entirely true. One guy felt so good about his progress (24 pounds lost and still going), he gave himself a complete makeover: new haircut, goatee, earring. But his motivation had nothing to do with his photo shoot.

Now, we'll admit this wasn't the most scientific of studies. For one thing, we didn't even measure testosterone. If that sounds like a surprising omission, just hear us out: Testosterone levels, like levels of most body chemicals, are constantly in flux. They can be affected by numerous variables beyond what a guy eats and lifts. And they're tricky to measure under the best of circumstances. Unless we took the guys in as boarders, monitoring everything they did, there was no way we could get testosterone values that would have any clinical significance. The last thing we wanted was to come up with data that confused the issue. So in this one case, we opted to fall back on those other clinical studies we cite throughout the book.

We don't think it's a major shortcoming, especially since we have observable evidence of the flab our guys lost, the muscle they gained, and the other, more subjective benefits they reported. The bottom line is, we got results. *Dramatic* results. That's what mattered to them, and we figure it's what matters to you.

Here's just the first of several success stories we'll feature throughout the book in "Before & After" profiles. We hope Cory and the rest of our guys inspire you to kick your own Testosterone Advantage Plan into high gear.

Around here, we called Cory Schmaldinst our poster boy—and we're not the only ones who've noticed his transformation.

Cory on the new him: "I haven't been at my current weight since college. And even then, I never looked like this."

On others' reactions: "People are shocked. They say, 'How long did it take?' I tell them 9 weeks, and they ask me, 'Where do I get this diet?'"

On the intangible results: "It changes you mentally too. I'm happier with myself. I have energy, and I feel I can do whatever I want."

On the T plan versus his past fitness efforts: "I'd run 3 or 4 days a week, and it wasn't getting me anywhere. I just figured it wasn't meant to be. Like my genes were wrong. . . . I tried Atkins, but you can't keep up with it. This diet is normal eating. It's a program you can stick to."

On his fiancée's reaction: "She definitely likes the way I look. Now, because I'm starting to look better, she's feeling the urge to get back to the gym. . . . Before, [my unhappiness] would affect our relationship. We get along so well now."

On his goals for the future: "I want my kids to say to their friends, 'You should see my dad.' I want to look good and not have problems when I'm 40."

Bottom line: "My life is so much easier. I'm happy with my body and my whole health picture."

CORY SCHMALDINST, 26, 6'

VITAL STATS		BEFORE T PLAN	AFTER T PLAN
	WEIGHT	190 lb	172 lb
	WAIST	36¾"	32"
	BENCH PRESS	215 lb	245 lb
	CHINUPS	7	"almost 13"

FIT OR MISFIT?

Picture two Olympic athletes. Both are extremely lean, with body-fat percentages in the low single digits. One guy's body is exactly what you'd visualize when you read the words *Olympic* and *athlete* in the same sentence: broad shoulders, narrow waist, thick arms, legs that look like they could kick a football 90 yards and catch up to it before it hit the ground. The other looks as if he were in the final stages of a tragic illness. You want to feed him, but you're not sure he could keep anything down.

As you've probably guessed, the first athlete is a sprinter, a man who never does traditional aerobic exercise and might not be able to run a mile without breaking it up into four quarter-mile dashes. The second is a marathoner, a guy who does nothing but aerobic exercise and might not be able to complete a single chinup or bench-press half his weight.

Of these two guys—one who appears to be ready to keel over, the other who looks like he had sex five times before breakfast—which one would you consider "fit"?

Easy question. Too easy. But we ask it for a reason. If you didn't have visual descriptions, if all you knew about these two guys were their aerobic-fitness levels, you would've said the gaunt marathoner was the most fit of the two.

And that's the crux of the problem we have with fitness as it's peddled in America. Given a choice, you'd rather look like the sprinter. And you're pretty sure the women you know would rather sleep with the sprinter. (What woman wants a guy who's skinnier than she is?) But the American fitness establishment wants you to train like the marathoner.

Oh, here's one more image to keep in mind, about the very origins of the word *marathoner*: According to legend, when the Greeks defeated the Persians in the battle of Marathon in 490 B.C., a runner named Pheidippides was dispatched to carry the good news back to Athens. At the end of his 22-mile journey, he reportedly shouted, "Rejoice! We conquer!"

And then he died of exhaustion.

THE BODY YOU WANT, IN THE TIME YOU HAVE

Traditional weight-control theory has given the chunky flunky three options: Eat fewer calories or burn more or some combination thereof.

Burning more calories is usually thought of as an active process, like jogging, lifting weights, or yanking your daughter out of some teenage Romeo's Mustang. But the majority of the calories you burn throughout the day are controlled by your basal metabolism. These are the calories your body burns whether you're active or not, whether you're sleeping or eating, whether you're thinking about sex or actually having some. Your body burns these calories to provide fuel for your brain, your heart, your other organs; to keep your muscles and other moving parts prepared for action.

Your body burns about 10 percent of its calories by digesting the food you eat, which is called the thermic effect of feeding. *Thermic* is a great word to remember, because it reminds you that your body is just one skin-wrapped furnace and that the food you eat is the fuel you feed your furnace.

The other—and most variable—way in which you burn calories is through voluntary activity. Exercising, playing with the kids, working in the yard, walking to the john—every move you make expends more calories than you would burn by just sitting still. Physical activity accounts for anywhere from 10 to 30 percent of the energy your body uses each day.

So let's review: Your body has three mechanisms for burning calories. Two of them you don't think about, because basal metabolism and the thermic effect of feeding are invisible to you. And yet, those two account for 70 to 90 percent of the fuel you burn each day. So it makes sense that the best way to control body weight is to ramp up those two systems. Build muscle, and you increase your metabolism by up to 50 calories a day per pound of muscle. Eat more protein, and you crank up the thermic effect by as much as one-third. (We'll do the math in chapter 6.) In effect, you achieve truly metabolic weight control: Fat burning that hums along on its own even as you sit or sleep or just stew about pulling your daughter out of some teenage Romeo's Mustang.

So what does the current paradigm for exercise and nutrition offer you? Exercise routines that not only fail to build more metabolism-boosting muscle but also reduce the muscle you already have. And diet programs that not only fail to take advantage of the thermic effect of protein but also lower your muscle-building testosterone by reducing the fat that provides the building blocks for your manliest hormone. This is the equivalent of sending soldiers into battle without bullets in their guns.

The one effective weapon the established guidelines do give you is activity. We agree that activity is important, and all of the authors of this book have a lifelong passion for strenuous exercise. But we have to admit that increasing activity is the slowest, most frustrating way to lose weight.

THE SPEED BURNERS

What we're going to give you in this book is the fastest, most sure-fire way to lose fat, gain muscle, restore your body to its natural athletic shape, and reinforce your vital male essence. The key is to tap naturally into your body's supply of testosterone, the male hormone that, to varying degrees, governs musculature, height, bone density, sexual function, and a host of other elements that are of critical importance to men.

You also need to know as much as possible about regulating other key self-made chemicals, like growth hormone and cortisol.

Our premise is simple: We've taken everything we now know about naturally boosting hormone levels and organized that information into a comprehensive eating-and-workout plan that you can put into effect on an individualized basis. Testosterone helps you maximize your muscle mass and mobilize fat for energy—in short, it helps you get the most out of your workouts. And if you follow our plan religiously—doing the right exercises in the right combinations at the right times—you'll spur your body's production of additional testosterone that will enable you to work out harder and longer and will aid your muscles in recovery and growth.

In a nutshell, the Testosterone Advantage Plan will allow you to adjust your body composition in order to meet your personal goals. You may want to drop 10 pounds of fat from around your waist. Or you may want to gain 10 pounds of muscle on your arms, legs, and chest. Whatever your specific goals are, we think that we can help you achieve them in a way that's impossible to do with any of those one-size-fits-all diets.

Are you going to miraculously transform yourself into one of those hulking figures you see on the cover of *Muscle & Fitness* magazine? No. Those guys have to commit their lives to looking that way. And many of them—probably most of them—are able to achieve their results only by injecting synthetic substances into their bodies. (Besides, research has shown that women don't necessarily lust after those types of bodies anyway. They prefer a lean, muscular look to a superhuman torso.)

But will the Testosterone Advantage Plan make you look better and feel better? Yes. Are you going to become the best *you* that you can be? We like to think so. And we're supported in this conviction by cutting-edge scientific research as well as the results of our own pilot program.

Although some of our concepts have been practiced in the world of bodybuilding for decades, the science underlying our plan is just starting to gain acceptance in the halls of academia. And when we say "academia," we're not talking about Hercules Tech. For example, the Harvard School of Public Health has conducted one of several major studies whose findings suggest that a high-fat, low-fiber diet raises testosterone levels.

We've organized these landmark insights into a simple 9-week plan, and we're confident that if you put it to work for you, you'll not only look and feel better but also become stronger than you've ever been and leaner than you've been since the days when you didn't even realize that it was a good shape to be in. Though your metamorphosis won't exactly be instant, you'll start getting measurably stronger after the first few workouts. Within 4 weeks, your body will start making important molecular adaptations that set the stage for gains in muscle size. After that, you could see muscle growth of 20 to 40 percent. Granted, those gains won't all happen in 9 weeks, but the foundation you build with this program will put you on the straightest, surest path to that destination.

And the best part of our program: You'll get to eat like a man and look like a god.

We believe we're ushering in an exciting new era in weight management for men. We're inviting you to join us on the frontier.

CHAPTER

2

Why Almost Everything You Know about Fitness Is Probably Dead Wrong

*A*s we've already suggested, when we men say that we want to "lose weight," generally what we mean is that we want to look better. We don't necessarily want to lose weight per se; we want to lose only the useless, unattractive weight, otherwise known as fat. We want less flab, more definition. And we want to get and stay fit. Those are important distinctions to make.

First of all, though we question many things in this book, the benefits of having a lean, fit body aren't among them (hence the "almost" in the title of this chapter). Let's take a side trip for a few moments to review what science—the new as well as the old—tells us fitness and fat loss can do for you.

YOU'LL LIVE LONGER

Let us say this in a more eye-catching fashion: You'll likely *die sooner* if you *don't* worry about fat or fitness. One landmark study of more than 755,000 people found that men who are 50 percent overweight are twice as likely to die prematurely as average-weight guys are.

Further, a study of more than 325,000 people, published in 1999 in the *American Journal of Epidemiology*, showed that among those ages 40 to 50, obesity increases the risk of death to that of a person 5.9 years older.

What, specifically, is likely to kill you if you're fat? Let's take a look.

HEART DISEASE AND STROKE remain the leading causes of death and permanent disability in men. The most serious problem with such conditions is that the first symptom may be death—which, historically, is hard to treat. Even if you don't actually keel over, being overweight contributes to the lesser condition of angina, a constricting chest discomfort caused by decreased oxygen flow to the heart. Overweight, unfit men are also far more likely to have two of the most important causative factors for heart disease and stroke: high blood pressure and elevated levels of "bad" cholesterol and blood fats called triglycerides.

Blood pressure, the force of flowing blood against your artery walls, is measured in two numbers, as in 120/80 (said as "120 over 80"). The 120, or systolic pressure, reflects the force used by the heart to pump blood through your body. The 80 is the ambient pressure in the arteries when your heart is at rest between pumps.

As many as 50 million Americans either currently have high blood pressure or take medication to remedy the condition. At least until late middle age, men are more likely victims than women. In both sexes, blood pressure tends to rise gradually with age. Allowed to go unchecked, high blood pressure makes you seven times more likely to have a stroke, six times more likely to develop congestive heart failure, and three times more likely to be a candidate for a heart attack. Long-term high blood pressure also causes kidney damage and blindness.

Even modest loss of flab can lower your blood pressure. In one 3-year study of 1,191 participants, researchers sought to quantify the long-term beneficial effects of fat loss on blood pressure. Subjects who lost weight lowered their systolic and diastolic blood pressures by as much as five and seven points, respectively, and lowered their risk of high blood pressure by 35 percent.

CANCER is the second most common cause of death, and fitness is increasingly being studied as a possible safeguard against it. This much does seem clear: Flabby, out-of-shape men more frequently develop cancers of the colon, rectum, and prostate. The American Cancer Society tells us that grossly overweight men are about 1.4 times more likely than lean men to develop these cancers.

Two studies presented at a recent annual meeting of the American College of Sports Medicine add to the mounting evidence that men with high fitness levels are less likely to die of cancer. One test that surveyed health patterns in some 22,703 men of various ages showed that men classified as unfit were 80 percent more likely to die of cancer than their fit counterparts were. Being a couch potato seemed to increase the risk of lung cancer in particular.

Now, this may be an example of dubious research, as the study seemed to ignore the fact that men who exercise more *also* are likely to be more health-conscious on the whole. Thus, they may have better eating habits and—we suspect—be far less likely to smoke. They may also visit their doctors more often, so the cancer is diagnosed and treated at an earlier stage. All of this means we're hard put to single out exercise or body-fat loss as the key factor in the fit-men's success against cancer. But the study is still food for thought—especially when combined with a separate study, reported in *The New England Journal of Medicine*, that argues that genetic factors may account for between 21 and 42 percent of cancer risk, with lifestyle and other factors accounting for the rest.

Overweight people are twice as likely to develop **DIABETES TYPE 2** (also called noninsulin-dependent diabetes mellitus) as people who are not overweight. The most common form of diabetes in the United States, this disease is a major cause of impotence, early death, heart disease, kidney disease, stroke, and blindness.

Then there's **ASTHMA**. Recent research proves that being overweight may actually be a causative factor for this ailment. A study of more than 85,000 women found that weight gain after age 18 significantly increased the risk of developing asthma.

"Being overweight is like having a constrictive jacket strapped across your chest," Joshua Needleman, M.D., assistant professor of pulmonary medicine at the Bronx-based Montefiore Medical Center, told CNN. "It squeezes your lungs, making them unable to function. It also pinches the breathing tubes."

A combination of extra body fat and too little exercise ups the risk of various bone disorders. A condition called **OSTEOARTHRITIS** places extra pressure on joints in the knees, hips, and lower back; it also wears down the cartilage that normally cushions and protects those joints. Fat loss decreases stress on the joints and may reduce the symptoms of existing disease.

A second "osteo"—**OSTEOPOROSIS**—has long been associated with aging women. And granted, four out of five people with the condition are women. But that still means one in five is a man. In fact, one out of every eight men over age 50 will suffer a bone fracture due to osteoporosis—surprisingly enough, for the same reason his wife might: lack of estrogen. Certain bone cells actually transform men's testosterone (hey, there's that hormone again) to estrogen, but the number of those cells and, hence, the amount of estrogen diminish with age. Men get osteoporosis 10 to 15 years later than women do because their drop in estrogen and bone density is more gradual. How does all of this relate to fitness? High-impact exercise such as weight lifting helps build the bone density that prevents osteoporosis.

Here's another malady to add to the list of skeletal problems: a type of arthritis known as **GOUT**. In this condition, crystals of a waste product called uric acid are deposited in joints, causing pain, swelling, and stiffness. (Curiously, about half of all cases affect the big toe.) Gout is more common in men than in women, and like every other ailment we've talked about, it's also more common in overweight people.

Finally, add **GALLBLADDER DISEASE** to the list of ailments for which you increase your risk if you're out of shape. Your risk increases proportionally with your weight gain.

Of course, many of these diseases are interrelated and have an unfortunate multiplier effect: Diabetes, for example, intensifies your risk for heart disease. So you're really betting against the house by doing nothing about fat and fitness.

But fitness isn't all about preventing disease and postponing death. There are obvious quality-of-life issues too.

"WASN'T HUNGRY AT ALL"

Ed Stash is the embodiment of the problem with homemade workout programs and so-called healthy diets. They don't work.

On life before the T plan: "*I was lifting weights every day, close to an hour and a half a day. I was also trying to keep in shape by eating low-fat foods. I thought I was watching what I ate, but it turns out I was probably taking in 1,000 calories a day that were a total waste. I was on this diet for 3 years and I worked out religiously. In those 3 years, I went up two pants sizes.*"

On the T diet: "*I wasn't hungry at all. There was more than enough food.*"

On physical results: "*I am the strongest I've ever been in my life. I got the greatest increases in strength in my biceps and triceps and in my back. I had to go out and buy a whole new wardrobe.*"

On others' reactions: "*People who hadn't seen me in a couple of months were shocked—a jaw-dropping reaction. When I was home visiting my parents, I saw a neighbor who was 20 or 21 years old. She hadn't seen me in about 8 years. She just came right out and said, 'You have a very nice ass.'*"

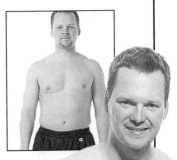

On his newfound vitality: "*My performance has gotten better at work. I get more done, [and] I'm not relying on anything artificial to keep me going. I just have natural energy that lasts throughout the day.*"

Bottom line: "*I feel more confident everywhere I go. Just seeing what I was able to accomplish, I feel better about myself.*"

ED STASH, 28, 5' 10"

VITAL STATS		BEFORE T PLAN	AFTER T PLAN
	WEIGHT	187 lb	172 lb
	WAIST	35"	32"
	CHINUPS	8	11

YOU'LL LIVE BETTER

The catalog of quality-of-life benefits is almost as impressive as the direct health benefits. For starters, you'll stay stronger longer. Lie around like a lump now, and before you know it, you may become a lump. Failure to commit a reasonable amount of time to fitness and strength building eventually can leave you too weak to do even basic household chores. Further, if you've been a slacker since day one, decrepitude may hit you much earlier in life than it should.

A study by the University of South Carolina's School of Public Health and the Cooper Institute for Aerobics Research suggests that sedentary middle-aged men start experiencing problems usually associated with senior citizens. Researchers followed 3,069 men and 589 women, ages 30 to 82, for an average of 5 years. The subjects were given ratings from zero to 6 (6 being the best) based on upper- and lower-body strength. At the follow-up, the 5's and 6's were far less likely to report problems with their recreational, household, and personal-care activities (ranging from cooking and getting dressed to scrubbing floors and walking up 10 stairs without resting). The high-strength men were about half as likely to report functional problems as the goof-offs.

Although such limitations are most common in older people, "the association between muscular strength and endurance and the subsequent prevalence of functional limitations indicates that this relationship persists even among middle-aged adults," said the report. In English, that means if you don't work to keep yourself in shape, you might fall apart long before you reach retirement age.

The good news is, it's never too late to start improving your body. Guys in their 50s who embark on a solid fitness program can reverse much of the damage that we've traditionally blamed on getting old, including declines in muscle strength, flexibility, energy level, and balance.

You'll also work **SMARTER**. In our hunt for weight-management solutions, we tend to overlook the degree to which a muscular physique promotes its own self-sustaining fitness advantages. Muscle mass requires nourishment. Equip your body with muscles, and more energy must be earmarked for maintaining those muscles. That's energy that, in less muscular people, simply becomes fat. You can eat more, once you get the muscles built. As long as you keep exercising, you keep the cycle going.

When it's time to rest, you'll **SLEEP BETTER**. Higher body weights increase your risk for sleep apnea, a serious condition marked by a cessation of breathing for short periods during sleep. Aside from causing you to awaken abruptly several times during the night (which makes you less likely to enjoy a good night's sleep), the condition often causes sufferers to snore heavily (which makes you more likely to sleep alone). It's also associated with high blood pressure, stroke, and heart failure.

Last but never least, you'll reap more **MONEY and SEX**. We're going to go way out on a limb here and assume you like both of these things. Studies have shown that a svelte guy earns more than his fatter counterpart does and that—here's a shocker—the lean, better-looking guy also hooks up with more women.

Technically, say experts, he doesn't get the girls because of his looks: Women rate income higher than good looks, as a 1997 UCLA survey of 3,407 adults suggests (and as the fabled sex lives of Henry Kissinger and Mick Jagger seem to confirm). Still, it works out to the same thing, because—as other studies tell us—tall, attractive men earn up to 10 percent more than their shorter, less attractive colleagues. Though the most recent investigations of this phenomenon took place in England and Poland, we're betting things work pretty much the same in your neighborhood. And yes, people actually study these things. The English researchers, for example, interviewed 11,000 33-year-olds of various shapes and sizes.

Now, we know you can't do much about your height. What you *can* change is whether or not women perceive you as attractive. It helps to lose the flab and to have your clothes fit right.

And fitness, we may as well mention, won't hurt your performance in the bedroom, either.

"Okay, you convinced me. I definitely want to get in shape. That means exercising for 30 minutes a day, three to five times a week. Right?"

Let's back up a minute.

When a man decides he doesn't like the way he looks, he usually describes himself as "overweight" or "out of shape." Thus, he tends to de-scribe his exercise goals in those same terms: to "lose weight and get in shape." You almost never hear a guy say he's going to "get fit." Fitness, to men, is an abstraction. We understand that there are health benefits to fitness, but for most of us it's an afterthought—something that "just sorta happens" along with the visible improvements.

So if lately you've been seeing a pasty mudslide where you once had a waistline—if that's why you bought this book—you're thinking primarily about changing the shape of your body. Everything else you'll get out of that reshaping—less chance of heart disease or stroke or adult-onset diabetes or any number of cancers—is likely a bonus to you. First and foremost, you want to get rid of that damned gut.

Now, the conventional prescription for the out-of-shape man is to go on a diet and to exercise—exercise aerobically, that is. On the surface, this even seems to make sense since a steady aerobic activity such as running burns more calories minute-for-minute than weight lifting or start-stop sports like tennis and basketball. And of course, as we've all been told again and again, you need extended periods of exercise in order to get the most out of those invisible health benefits. Right?

Not so fast.

Ten years ago, the *American Journal of Cardiology* caused something of a furor, which included irking the hell out of a lot of the aerobic-exercise establishment. The journal's great sin was to pose that you didn't need to follow the recommended "20 minutes a day, 3 or 4 days a week" model in order to get a definable benefit from exercising.

Then in 2000, the American Heart Association published a study indicating that two 15-minute exercise sessions curb heart-disease risk as much as a single 30-minute session does. The researchers reviewed data on 7,307 men from 1988 through 1993. The men reported their exercise in as little as 15-minute segments. As long as the energy they expended was the same, it didn't matter whether they did their exercise in several shorter bouts or in one longer segment.

An 18-month study published in 1999 in the *Journal of the American Medical Association* also indicated that short bouts of exercise scattered throughout the day or week offered weight-loss and fitness benefits comparable to those achieved in much longer, continuous workout sessions.

"We know that there's a threshold level of activity needed to gain health benefits, but it's not necessary to get all this activity at one time," was the word from the study's lead author, John M. Jakicic, Ph.D., an assistant professor of research in the department of psychiatry and human behavior at the Brown University School of Medicine in Rhode Island.

We know what you're thinking. . . .

"So what's the lowest level of exercise I need?"

Meet Glenn A. Gaesser, a professor of exercise physiology at the University of Virginia and co-author of *The Spark: The Revolutionary 3-Week Fitness Plan That Changes Everything You Know about Exercise, Weight Control, and Health.* (And no, we're not thrilled about touting a competing author, but in this book we're going to call it as we see it.) Gaesser combined 10-minute exercise periods with a sensible eating plan and tested the program on 40 sedentary people. On average, in 3 weeks, participants lost a respectable 3 pounds, boosted their aerobic capacity by as much as 15 percent, showed strength and endurance increases ranging from 40 percent to 100 percent, significantly improved flexibility scores, cut their total cholesterol by as much as 34 points, and reduced their risk of heart disease by up to 40 percent.

"So then, 10 minutes is the lower limit? I couldn't do 20 separate 'workouts' of 1 minute a piece instead of the traditionally recommended 20-minute block of time—that'd be crazy, right?"

Well, maybe not. A study published in *Preventive Medicine* suggests that walking bouts of only 5 minutes—when they add up to 30 minutes a day, most days of the week—can pay some dividends in cardiovascular health and body composition.

This may be welcome news, especially if one of your excuses for not exercising is that you don't have time. It's estimated that a mere 15 percent of us comply with the American College of Sports Medicine's prescribed fitness regimen for adults. That daunting regimen calls for 20 to 45 minutes of aerobic exercise in your "target heart-rate zone," 3 to 5 days a week, plus strengthening and flexibility exercises 2 or more days a week. That doesn't leave too many days out.

But we'll tell you right up front, it's not as if you won't have to get off your duff and invest some effort in the T program. You do realize that, right? Our workouts *will* demand a reasonable amount of time.

"So why even mention all these studies?"

Simple. Our point is that medical science gradually and grudgingly has been coming around to the realization that short, intense bursts of exercise—exactly like those we've designed for you—offer health benefits previously identified with more sustained, aerobic exercise. And in a way, that shouldn't surprise anyone, since some of the earliest studies linking activity and lifespan weren't at all about jogging or cycling. In the early 1950s, Stanford epidemiologist Ralph Paffenbarger began a 22-year study of longshoremen in San Francisco and showed that the men who did the physical work had lower risk of cardiovascular disease than their desk-bound supervisors. In other words, being physically active is better for your health than being a slug. Nothing earthshaking there.

Later, though, Paffenbarger was instrumental in launching the Harvard Alumni Health Study, which looked at the physical activity of 12,516 middle-aged men from 1977 to 1993 and found that men who expended at least 1,000 calories a week in physical activity had about a 20-percent reduction in heart-disease risk. But men who expended 1,000 to 2,000 calories a week in *vigorous* exercise had a *30* percent lower risk of dying from *any* cause. The study defined "vigorous" exercise as equal to or greater than six metabolic units, or "mets."

In the T workout program, you'll burn more than 1,000 total calories per week, all of which will be in an activity above six mets. In fact, let's get this straight right here: Weight lifting provides enough exercise at a high-enough intensity to protect your heart and extend your life.

You may be wondering how we can be so forthright in proclaiming such heresy. What about that chorus loudly and persistently singing the praises of aerobic exercise? What about all those health organizations with the fancy acronyms? Is it possible that they're all wrong?

We'll just say this: If you came of age on the notion that jogging could one day save your life, prepare yourself for a big-time shock.

CHAPTER

3

The
Cardio
Conundrum

We like the word *conundrum*. (We also like *cavitation*, but we had a hard time working it into this book.) *Conundrum* is the perfect word, maybe the only word, for what we're going to talk about in this chapter.

We believe that any exercise is better than none. And we'll acknowledge, right here at the start of the chapter, that decades of solid science have shown an association between endurance exercises such as running and an impressive-sounding list of benefits: weight control, heart health, disease prevention, and the most important one of all, increased life span.

But if you're a committed runner, you may want to brace yourself: You're about to run up against some blunt facts.

FACT: The correlation between outward fitness and internal coronary health is tenuous. You can be a walking mass of plugged-up arteries and still be able to perform feats of exceptional "fitness"—till one day you suddenly drop dead while eating lasagna. Or, if you're jogging pioneer Jim Fixx, while jogging. At the ripe old age of 52.

Indeed, taken to extremes, aerobics can enlarge your heart, a particularly dangerous condition if you also have undiagnosed arterial disease, according to New York City cardiologist Henry Solomon, author of *The Exercise Myth*. Further, Dr. Solomon also believes that a fanatical devotion to intense aerobic exercise can lead to temporary or even long-term heart-rhythm disturbances. In his experience, overzealous runners often need pacemakers in their later years.

FACT: Aerobic exercise has been oversold as a one-stop-shop for better health. As noted, the health benefits of aerobic exercise can largely be achieved with any physical activity, whether it's at work, around the house, in the weight room—even in the bedroom, if you're vigorous enough about it. Aerobic exercise also is an overrated tool for weight control. Although it burns more calories than strength training while you're actually doing it, it can also decrease muscle mass and thus slow down your metabolism, which ultimately leads to weight regain.

FACT: Heart health aside, aerobic activities are more dangerous than the public has been led to believe. Among people over age 35, bicycling and running lead to some 85,000 more emergency-room visits than weight lifting does, according to the U.S. Consumer Product Safety Commission. And "runner's knee" is the most common chronic exercise injury, according to the Cooper Institute for Aerobics Research, despite the fact that running ranks only fifth on the list of the most popular exercise activities (weight lifting is number one). What's more—or maybe in this case what's less—aerobic exercise does little to prepare your body for sports activities. Most sports involve quick bursts of activity and sudden changes of direction. Slow, steady endurance exercise merely trains your body to become good at moving slowly and steadily.

OBSERVATION + FACT: If aerobic exercise truly produced heart health, common sense says the benefits of such conditioning should transfer from one sport to another. This doesn't happen. Take the case of a weekend athlete who, on July 1, can run 3 miles or swim 10 laps before he's so completely winded that he has to quit. If he spends the next 3 months working only on his running, on October 1 he may very well be able to run 5 miles before exhaustion sets in. But in all likelihood, he'll *still be able to do only the same, original 10 laps in the pool*, or perhaps one or two more, before getting winded. Strange but true. The implication here? What that weekend athlete is really training between July 1 and October 1 is not his heart but the specific muscles enabling him to do his running. Plus, he's no doubt making adaptations in his running style that allow him to sprint more efficiently.

Is aerobics starting to sound a bit less like the godsend it was supposed to be?

A SHORT COURSE IN EXERCISE PHYSIOLOGY

Exercise is described as either aerobic or anaerobic. Weight training generally has been lumped in the latter category, as anaerobic, though the border between the two types of exercise is not quite so cut-and-dried as many would have you believe.

Using traditional definitions, words like *aerobic* and *cardio* tend to be reserved for sustained physical activities that are intense enough to significantly increase your body's oxygen consumption. Essentially, they make you huff and puff. The textbook examples would be jogging, cycling, swimming, kickboxing, treadmill work, and so forth. (So yes, sex is aerobic, provided you last more than a few minutes.) These are the sorts of activities the American Heart Association and similar groups have in mind when they say, "You need to exercise."

Your body generally calls upon three different substances to fuel itself during exercise: glycogen (that's the stored form of carbohydrate), fat, and, in some circumstances, protein. The primary fuels during aerobic exercise are fat (from body tissue as well as from sources within the muscles themselves) and carbohydrate (muscle glycogen and blood sugar). Low-intensity aerobic exercise relies almost entirely on fat for fuel.

As exercise intensity increases, your body gradually switches over

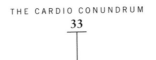

from fat and glycogen to glycogen alone. This point more or less corresponds with something called the lactate threshold. Push past this threshold and—if you've done much vigorous exercise you know what we're about to say—you become intimately familiar with The Burn that flares up from the accumulation of lactic acid in the muscles you're overtaxing.

The increase in glycogen use at higher exercise intensities is driven by a number of factors, including the release of adrenaline, your muscles' inability to get the energy they need from the quantity of fatty acids circulating in your blood, and the greater involvement of different types of muscle fibers.

When aerobic exercise continues at fairly intense (but not full-out) levels, or even at less intense levels but for extended periods, your system drifts into what's known as depletion: You exhaust your first-tier energy sources (that is, your glycogen stores) and actually begin metabolizing yourself: "eating up" muscle tissue to convert that protein into the energy you need to keep on going. Researchers have known for a while that once the body reaches this plateau, it burns up 5 to 6 grams of protein for every 30 minutes of ongoing activity.

This muscle loss is magnified if you're on a low-calorie diet while you're doing all this aerobic exercise, and magnified *further* if your diet follows the stingy protein recommendations in the U.S. dietary guidelines: 0.8 gram per kilogram of body weight, or 73 grams a day for a 200-pound man.

All of this is exacerbated as you age, because in your early 30s, you begin losing 1 to 2 percent of muscle mass each year anyway—a 5- to 10-pound loss of muscle per decade.

MULLING OVER MAX

We've said that aerobic exercise confers a number of health benefits, all of which can also be derived from other types of physical activity. The greatest health benefit, of course, is lack of death, and it has been generally assumed that only aerobic exercise adds years to your life. That's why researchers were surprised to learn in 1988 that increased aerobic fitness produces a significant decrease in mortality only in people who start out as complete slugs.

That study, presented at the annual meeting of the American College of Sports Medicine, looked at more than 10,000 men and classified them in five categories according to aerobic fitness. The least fit quintile (*quintile*, like *conundrum*, being one of those words we can't pass up a chance to use) had a death rate of 64 per 10,000. The second-worst quintile had a death rate of 25.5. And get this: The middle aerobic quintile had a death rate that was slightly *higher* than the second-worst group: 27.1.

Granted, the fittest group had the lowest death rate (18.6 per 10,000), but the researchers concluded that the only significant protection from all-cause mortality came from improvement in the least-fit group—the one that went from "I get winded when I walk from the couch to the refrigerator" to "I can walk around the block a couple of times."

The measure used to determine fitness in this study—and the standard we generally refer to when we discuss aerobic fitness—is VO_2 max. This is usually determined by a treadmill test, and it tells you how much oxygen you can consume per milliliter of blood. The more oxygen you can pull into your lungs and thus into your bloodstream, the harder your body can work.

VO_2 max is, to a large extent, inherited. Estimates on the degree to which it's genetic vary wildly, from 25 percent on up. A 1999 study in the *Journal of Applied Physiology* put 481 people from multiple generations of 98 families through a 20-week training program and concluded that the VO_2 max response to exercise is about 47 percent familial, with 28 percent coming from the mother's gene pool. Baseline VO_2 max—the aerobic-fitness levels before starting the program—showed an even higher genetic basis: 59 percent, with 36 percent maternal. So if you want your children to become elite endurance athletes, your best strategy is to marry an elite endurance athlete.

So we know VO_2 max is largely genetic and only marginally associated with longevity. And this leads to the biggest questions of all: Why should anyone care about aerobic fitness? What real benefits come from improved aerobic capacity that wouldn't arise from any other type of physical activity?

First off, improving your aerobic capacity improves your ability to perform endurance exercise. But you still improve only in the specific endurance exercise you practice. Remember the weekend athlete we mentioned earlier in this chapter, who after a 3-month running program added 2 miles to his running endurance threshold yet could swim, at most, only one or two additional laps before getting winded? That example illustrates that the most significant adaptations to aerobic exercise occur in the specific muscles being exercised. Those muscles become more efficient at using oxygen to convert carbohydrate and fat to energy—and that's a terrific benefit. But it's also a benefit you can achieve doing other types of activity.

Another way to improve VO_2 max is to lose weight. A man who loses more than 20 pounds may see his aerobic fitness improve by 10 percent—without doing any aerobic exercise. Do his heart and lungs become more efficient? No; he has less body mass, so the same amount of oxygen is used by a smaller body, increasing his "fitness" level.

A final thought about the benefits of endurance exercise: Life and sports are lived in a 360-degree environment in which sudden bursts of exertion and quick expressions of muscular power are the norm. Most traditional aerobic exercise improves your ability to perform a slow, steady activity in a straight line over a long period of time—which resembles almost nothing you ask your body to do on a regular basis.

A SHORT HISTORY OF THE "AEROBICS MOVEMENT"

Given everything we've said so far in this chapter, you're probably wondering how "fitness" and "aerobic fitness" got so entwined. After all, the first studies linking activity and longevity weren't at all about

"SHE WANTS ME TO MODEL"

Though not our most impressive subject in pure strength terms, J. C. Kelleher underwent one of our most dramatic personal transformations.

On his reasons for trying the T plan: *"I was having problems with headaches and chest pains. I was lacking energy, wasn't able to keep up with my kids. I got winded easily. I had to buy pants that were bigger and bigger. I wasn't feeling real good about myself."*

On his past attempts at losing weight: *"I'd go faithfully to a gym and work out three or four times a week and see absolutely no results."*

On the T plan itself: *"I never felt empty. I made my meals the prior night, and I was dedicated to it."*

On his results: *"This is basically the least I've ever weighed as an adult. I'm doing a lot more with my kids. We'll play soccer or shoot hoops; I can maneuver around now like I couldn't before. I have more energy. I even stopped snoring. This past Friday, I had to go shopping for clothes—again! My children threw their arms around me, and a tear ran down my face as they saw me fit into size 36. I haven't been size 36 since I was 19."*

On his wife's reaction: *"Last night, she looked at me and said with a smile, 'I lost half my husband.' She wants me to model clothing for her. She checks me out in the dressing room as I'm changing. She wants me to turn around so she can see my backside. I have more 'quality time' with her."*

Bottom line: *"It changed my life."*

J.C. KELLEHER, 35, 5' 10"

VITAL STATS		BEFORE T PLAN	AFTER T PLAN
	WEIGHT	224 lb	199 lb
	WAIST	43"	38"

running or cycling. They simply showed that being active is better for your health than the alternative.

As scientists further investigated the connection between activity and health, they focused on aerobic exercise primarily because it was easy to focus on. Put a guy on a treadmill, stick a breathing tube in his mouth and a few electrodes on his chest, and voilà: instant research project. They could also study more long-term effects in a pretty quantifiable way since most people who ran regularly had a general idea how far they ran and how long it took them.

By the late 1970s, the aerobics ball was zooming merrily along, pushed by the very public advocacy of Dr. Kenneth Cooper, founder of the Cooper Aerobics Center in Dallas, and especially runner-author-guru Jim Fixx; his classic tome, *The Complete Book of Running*, sold a gazillion copies and single-handedly *elevated* the blood pressures of motorists across America by putting all those joggers out there on the side of the road. Cooper, Fixx, and their partisans in the medical community linked aerobic exercise to every health benefit imaginable: less body fat, less heart disease, fewer strokes, lower cholesterol.

Then in 1978, the American College of Sports Medicine issued its now-famous edicts about how much aerobic exercise every adult needed to get. And if you asked, they'd let you know that their recommendation was the minimum—you'd actually be far better off if you did more.

Anyone who challenged the need for aerobic exercise or made the case that strength training could yield many of the same benefits without the repetitive stress on muscles and joints was branded a flake—a dangerous one, at that.

Exit, in the summer of 1984, Jim Fixx. He collapsed and died while jogging on a backwoods Vermont road. An autopsy revealed massive coronary artery disease: Two of his arteries were almost completely blocked and a third was partially occluded. While the running community was shocked, doctors noted that Fixx had one of the strongest risk factors for heart disease: a family history. (His father had his first heart attack at age 35 and died at 43.) Fixx's death, of course, was just a single anecdotal event—one lone man dying on one lonely road. Still, the irony was hard to resist. And it raised a troubling question: If aerobic exercise couldn't keep its own spiritual leader alive, what did that mean for the rest of us?

THE LIFTERS FIGHT BACK

Post-Fixx, the exercise paradigm began to shift. Through the mid-1980s and into the '90s, strength training skyrocketed. By 1997, it had become the most popular fitness activity in the United States, overall participation having increased almost 90 percent since 1987. That surge in interest sparked new research. Doctors and clinicians began experimenting with strength training in cardiac rehabilitation. They were somewhat shocked to find that strength training significantly lowered several cardiac risk factors that were previously thought to be affected only by aerobics.

With all of this came a new challenge to the aerobics-first assumption, especially as it applied to men. Weight control traditionally had been regarded as a straightforward "eat less, exercise more" prescription. To that point, the "exercise more" part had consisted almost entirely of aerobics.

When researchers began comparing aerobic exercise with strength training, they found that aerobics was indeed effective for helping guys slim down. But much of the weight that men lost was muscle mass, so they tended to experience metabolic slowdowns since, once they stopped the actual exercise, their bodies no longer had to provide fuel for as much musculature. Thus, 230-pound Joe Average who used aerobics to help him slim down to 165 pounds ended up with a slower basal (resting) metabolism than a guy who'd been 165 his entire life. In order to hold on to his newly trim body, Joe would have to eat less than other 165-pounders—*possibly forever*. Because Joe was not capable of that kind of discipline, he almost inevitably regained the weight. And of course, because he wasn't lifting weights or otherwise challenging his muscles, the weight he regained was ugly, useless flab.

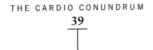

Researchers began to ask themselves: What if we switched things around? What if we took that same 230-pound guy and had him lift weights while restricting his dietary intake?

In short order, they made a series of interrelated, eye-opening discoveries.

1. Because the weight lifting wasn't as continuous an activity as the aerobics, Joe didn't burn as many calories, so he didn't lose as much weight per se. The good news: All the weight that he did lose was fat. He hung on to his muscle and even built new muscle.

2. Weight training *itself* spurred testosterone production. And certain types of training—particularly compound lifting that involved several major muscle groups working together—spurred it to a dramatic degree. Too much hard-core aerobic exercise, on the other hand, shut down T production.

3. Both aerobics and weight training resulted in immediate-aftermath metabolic increases. However, the metabolic effect of aerobics lasted only 30 minutes to an hour. The effect of weight training lasted anywhere from 30 minutes to as long as 48 hours. That's up to 48 hours during which the body metabolized fat, not muscle. As for basal metabolism, the weight trainer's actually increased rather than decreased, because his body now needed to support extra musculature (at the rate of up to 50 calories per day per pound of lean muscle, depending on variables).

So our friend Joe might get down to only 185 pounds, instead of 165, but his metabolism would run *faster* than that of a 185-pound jogger who was thin as a rail and couldn't lift a rail if his life depended on it. Plus, subjectively, Joe looked better than he did when he'd lost weight via aerobic exercise. And he had a better chance of keeping the weight off.

There is no minimizing the bottom-line implication here: The more muscle with which you equip your body, the easier it is for you to lose fat. Your body takes care of that on its own—your *metabolic* weight loss, remember?—simply by virtue of your stepped-up metabolism. Indeed, hard-core bodybuilders typically step up their eating just to sustain the same constant weight.

As the research continued, other myths began to fall, like poor Jim Fixx himself, by the wayside.

MYTH: "If I want to do both weight lifting and aerobics, I should do aerobics first."

Because aerobic exercise has been promoted as more "important" than strength training, it followed that guys who wanted to do both would start a workout with aerobics and only afterward proceed to the weight room. Even guys who gave equal importance to the two exercise modes thought that aerobic exercise would serve as a warmup for strength work, but that the converse wouldn't be true because if they lifted weights first, they'd be too tired to get an effective aerobic workout.

First off, the way to prepare your body for strength training is to perform strength exercises with a lower weight. Second, aerobic training before weight training can burn enough glycogen out of your muscle cells to make your weight workout ineffective. On the other hand, doing strength work before aerobic work can make the aerobics more effective. You start the exercise with less glycogen, so your body needs to rely more on fat from the get-go.

It is true that you should warm up in some fashion for strength exercise. You do need to increase your body's core temperature to make your lifting as productive as possible. If you want to spend 5 minutes on a treadmill to do that, fine. But you can warm up with any type of activity. And if it's a warm day and you're sweating before you open the gym door, you can go straight to the weight room and do your warmup sets of whatever exercise you're starting out with.

MYTH: "I need to be flexible. Weight lifting will make me muscle-bound."

Let's see, do you mean muscle-bound like Andre Agassi, who credits a strength-training program for his return to the pinnacle of the tennis world after a several-year lull (though dumping Brooke Shields may have helped)? Or maybe you mean muscle-bound like Mark McGwire, whose massive physique obviously hasn't robbed him of one of the game's quickest bats, which he uses to deposit hordes of 95-mph fast-balls into the bleachers of ballparks far and wide. For that matter, have you taken a good look at the chests and shoulders of our Olympic swimmers and gymnasts lately? Do their muscles seem to be inhibiting them?

Oh, and before you even worry about being flexible, you should first hope to avoid crippling yourself. Though weight lifting (like any physical activity) is not risk-free, herewith is a recent sampling of headlines from the world of aerobics.

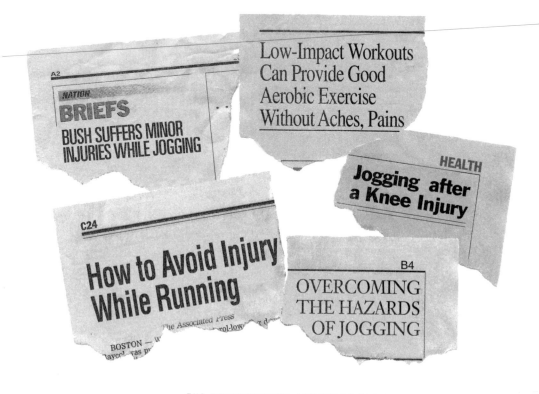

A2

NATION
BRIEFS
BUSH SUFFERS MINOR INJURIES WHILE JOGGING

Low-Impact Workouts Can Provide Good Aerobic Exercise Without Aches, Pains

HEALTH
Jogging after a Knee Injury

C24
How to Avoid Injury While Running
The Associated Press
BOSTON —

B4
OVERCOMING THE HAZARDS OF JOGGING

Even the godfather of aerobics himself, Dr. Cooper, suffered knee problems and chronic Achilles tendinitis after pounding the pavement for more than 20,000 miles. He has since added a knee-friendly rubberized jogging trail to his Dallas clinic complex and has cut back his personal running program to 15 miles a week. (Following Fixx's death, Cooper wrote a book entitled *Running without Fear: How to Reduce the Risk of Heart Attack and Sudden Death during Aerobic Exercise*.)

And let's not forget psychiatrist William Glasser, M.D., who in his landmark book, *Positive Addiction*, made note of the large number of guilt-wracked joggers and runners who continued to run, possibly to their physical detriment, even after tendinitis set in and their joints no doubt began to crumble. This in a book that set out to frame running as a worthwhile obsession. (For the record, strength training not only promotes bone density and reduces bone loss but also helps *rehabilitate* orthopedic injuries.)

And consider: When you lift weights in a gym or in your house, you're 100 percent less likely to get hit by a car than if you were out jogging.

MYTH: "But weight lifting does nothing for my heart!"

In 1990, the American College of Sports Medicine first recognized strength training as an important part of a complete exercise program for all healthy adults. A decade later, the American Heart Association issued an advisory in its own journal, *Circulation*, stating that strength training does in fact *improve* heart health. The AHA strongly recommended a weight-lifting program to prevent cardiovascular disease and to help rehabilitate those who have suffered mild heart attacks.

What prompted these groups to have a change of heart, so to speak, about the benefits of strength training? Research clearly had begun to show that weight lifting can provide modest bumps in VO_2 max (remember, this is a measure of your body's ability to process oxygen). Evidence also had come to light that regular strength training lowers resting blood pressure and levels of "bad" (LDL) cholesterol while enhancing your stroke volume (a sexy-sounding term for the amount of blood your heart pumps with each beat). In addition, studies found that strength training can decrease the stress on your heart when you do everyday tasks like carrying heavy trash bags to the curb, and that pumping iron improves your body's ability to respond to glucose. (Improved glucose tolerance prevents diabetes.) Further, research shows that weight lifting may even protect against damage by free radicals, naturally occurring, highly reactive molecules that can damage DNA and cause mutations that can lead to heart problems, stroke, and cancer.

Let's not forget, though, that we're going to show you how to use weight lifting to increase your testosterone production. And much new research links testosterone in its own right to a number of heart-healthy results.

In fact, maybe it's time we met this amazing substance up close and personal. . . .

CHAPTER

4

Testosterone:
A Man's Key
to Getting and Staying Fit

*I*n workout circles, it's called the juice, and for good reason. "It," of course, is testosterone. When bodybuilders use the term, they tend to refer to the injectable kind, or anabolic steroids (*anabolic* from the Greek for "to build"). For our purposes, we mean that definably male chemical your body produces entirely on its own.

For simplicity's sake, we're mostly going to call it T from here on.

According to the most recent research, your testes secrete T in a circadian manner, which is to say, on a regular cyclic schedule. Though no two men share the exact same T-production cycle, the rule of thumb is that T levels peak in the early morning. The daily erection that also peaks, for most of us, at about 5:00 A.M. helps one appreciate the very direct link between T and proper sexual function.

Although that last sentence alone may have sold you on the idea of trying to boost your T, we thought you might be interested in just a bit more background on the subject before we set about augmenting your natural supply of juice.

First, be aware that your body's production of T starts to drop off somewhere between your mid-20s and late 30s. The exact age is a matter of some debate. This much isn't: If you're our average reader—42ish—you're almost certainly on the downslope. Without intervention of some sort, you'll continue down that wistful hill for the rest of your life.

That's a damn shame, because nature clearly intended for you to make all-purpose use of T. Receptor sites exist in your brain, your heart, your nervous system, and elsewhere throughout your body, belying the oversimplified (and misleading) description of testosterone as a "sex hormone." Aside from the functions we're going to discuss here, T plays a role in your oxygen utilization, blood sugar balance, cholesterol regulation, immune system upkeep, and overall neurological function.

Within the fitness and medical communities, T's role in muscle building and overall body composition is beyond dispute. That doesn't change what we said at the outset of this book: We expect you to take nothing for granted. That's why we're going to outline just a few of the more convincing studies of T and its effects.

Realize that in the not-too-distant past, testosterone research tended to be something of a fringe pursuit. (And once again, we don't mean to sound like conspiracy theorists, but studies on the equivalent female hormone, estrogen, abound.) Even today, much of the work on testosterone is taking place at the cutting edge of science. This means that to make our case, we have to rely, to some degree, on inference and circumstantial evidence. That's not all bad. Sometimes common sense is as valuable as the so-called hard proof that medical science gives us, anyway. Decades ago, researchers gave us "hard proof" that we should switch from butter to margarine. Today, some of those same experts are telling us to switch back.

Realize, too, that almost all important scientific discoveries have begun with small pockets of anecdotal data. For example, in the early 1980s, doctors in urban centers on both coasts noticed that male patients were trickling in with a strange disorder that seemed to be zapping their immune systems and, often, causing strange red blotches on their faces and other parts of their bodies. The doctors took personal histories and learned that almost all of these patients were gay. As the early trend swelled into an alarming epidemic, doctors theorized—*based on the anecdotal information available to them to that point*—that some terrible new bug was afoot in the gay community. As months passed, having little else to go on, researchers further theorized that this new syndrome was spread by homosexual contact. This, of course, was medical science's first hazy awareness of the modern plague that more intensive research later diagnosed as the AIDS virus.

So in the spirit of blazing new trails, we present a sampling of interesting T-related studies from the past few years.

JUST THE FACTS, MAN

In one 1996 clinical trial, 43 men were divided into four groups, two of which received weekly 600-milligram injections of testosterone for 10 weeks, and two of which took placebo injections. The two T groups were then subdivided into those who worked out and those who basically sat back and waited for their T to kick in. Men in the latter group did reap gains in muscle size and strength, despite their relative lack of activity. But—and this will take on even greater significance for you very soon—it was the guys who also worked out who experienced the truly dramatic gains. By the end of the 10 weeks, each of them had added an average of 13 pounds of solid muscle and bench-pressed an extra 48 pounds.

Equally telling (and more body-part-specific) results were reported in 1999 by the School of Exercise Science and Sports Management at Southern Cross University in Lismore, Australia. Researchers recruited 21 weight-training subjects in a study to determine T's effects on body composition, upper-body strength, and overall health. Improvements in lean-tissue mass, arm girth, and thigh circumference were unmistakable for all volunteers taking T. Further—of particular interest to guys trying to lose unsightly guts—abdominal skin folds showed significant decreases in the testosterone group. (Though skin-fold measurements recently have lost favor among serious students of conditioning science, the test has been in common usage for many years and is a typical component of weight-control studies.)

In another study, this one published in 2000, researchers at the

Charles R. Drew University of Medicine and Science in Los Angeles combined T supplementation with strength training in HIV-infected men who were losing weight and had declining levels of natural T. Sixty-one subjects were split into four groups: placebo and no exercise; placebo plus weight training; supplemental T and no exercise; and T plus weight training. Each of the men given T added more than 5 pounds of muscle to his frail frame and displayed significant strength gains—even the guys who didn't lift a single dumbbell during the 34-month study. This suggests that T may be of special benefit to men whose health is compromised to begin with.

A study at one large Italian university looked at muscular responses to a single heavy-duty resistance-training session. Noting that muscle fibers in the men with higher T concentrations tended not to fatigue as quickly, the researchers concluded that the hormone somehow ensured better neuromuscular efficiency. This allowed the lucky guys to work out longer and harder, providing more ultimate bang for the buck in the same way that certain fuel additives are said to enable cars to get greater mileage out of the same quantity of gas.

How and why all this happens is still being investigated.

"Okay, so T works. But won't more of it make me meaner— and then kill me?"

If you're like most guys, what you've heard about testosterone to date hasn't been especially comforting. T has taken a lot of hits in the media for causing everything from "'roid rage" to heart disease. Once more, let's look a bit closer.

In the first study we mentioned above, the one involving 43 men, the only changes observed in the half who took T were positive; no mood or behavior differences were noted over the course of the entire 10-week program.

There does seem to be some anecdotal evidence of aggressiveness or moodiness in guys taking large doses of testosterone. However, there are two key points to consider. One is the phrase *large doses*. Indiscriminate self-dosing with T—which, make no mistake, is a potent chemical—is no less stupid and no more the fault of the substance itself than over-medication with a strong painkiller like codeine. You can't blame the codeine if you double up on the dosage, get behind the wheel of your car, and drift off the road in a medicated stupor. Similarly, it's not T's fault if some gym rat bent on becoming the next Schwarzenegger keeps jabbing himself in the buttock or thigh with reckless amounts of steroids.

Second, there's a definite distinction between the T that you inject and the T that you prompt your body to supply on its own. To return to the codeine analogy, it's like the difference between the adrenaline surge you get while pumping iron—which most of us would agree is beneficial and poses no danger—and the sort of high you get by gobbling little white pills. Your system is very good at self-regulating. Yes, you can spur your body into doing a little more of this or a little less of that, but always within boundaries set by nature. That's why we'll admit this right up front: No one should have any illusions about using our Testosterone Advantage Plan to get his body to *triple* its production of the stuff. That's not gonna happen, no matter how much fat you eat or how much exercise you do. In fact, after a certain point, overly strenuous or continuous exercise causes T levels to plummet. And a diet of 97 percent fat may be undesirable for other reasons (though in ensuing chapters, we're going to introduce you to some men who did well even on diets that were up to 70 percent fat!).

Scientific trials that have attempted to approximate the body's stepped-up production of T at biophysically realistic levels have yielded the good (the muscle mass and lean tissue) without any of the supposed bad stuff that somehow found its way into the popular consciousness. No sudden, rampant loss of hair. No acne outbreaks. No heart trouble.

Negative effects are likely, however, in someone who's operating at *deficient* levels of T. A guy with low T levels may have low libido (loss of interest in sex) and erectile problems (difficulty performing with the partners who do interest him). It stands to reason that correcting these morale-sapping problems should help make a man a happier camper.

This intuition gained credence in June 2000, when the makers of AndroGel topical T ointment reported the findings of a study of 227 men who'd volunteered to try the product under close supervision by doctors at the Harbor-UCLA Research and Education Institute. In addition to the tangible strength, muscle-mass, and bone-density gains clinicians expected, the men also showed distinct improvements in mood. The upshot? You can reassure your boss, your significant other, and the local authorities that our program won't transform you into a grunting Neanderthal. But when your significant other is in the mood for a very special kind of grunting, you'll be in better shape to oblige. (Oh, did we forget to mention that the men using the T gel also had improved sexual function as well?)

Let's turn to the other area where T has gotten a major public-relations black eye: heart health. This blemish no doubt stems from anecdotal horror stories of steroid-abusing bodybuilders who drop in mid-workout. Let's try to keep things in perspective. Sadly, some very robust-looking young men do keel over and die for no apparent reason; usually, autopsies reveal heart defects that have been ticking away like time bombs, often since birth. Or, as in the case of runner Jim Fixx, the casualties were in advanced stages of heart disease, despite their outwardly healthy appearance. And to the extent that overdoing T *can* perhaps cause adverse cardiological effects, be mindful again of the risks of self-medicating. Anything, taken to excess, can kill you.

Actually, recent clinical testing strongly suggests that, far from causing heart disease, testosterone delays its onset and lessens its adverse effects.

- In three separate studies in China, Turkey, and the United States, researchers administered quantities of T sufficient to raise the levels of their T-deficient older subjects to mid-normal. The results? All three studies showed substantially decreased total cholesterol and "bad" LDL cholesterol. The Chinese study also reported higher "good" HDL cholesterol.
- A study at a large London health-research facility showed that T exerts a relaxing, dilating effect on coronary arteries. It involved 13 men age 50 and older who were given physiological concentrations of T (which basically means they received dosages

"LIKE NEWLYWEDS AGAIN"

There was one particular side benefit of increased testosterone production that we'd been wondering about, and we're happy to report that Greg Kemler noticed it, alright. His wife may be less happy to see what he confesses below.

On his weight-loss epiphany: "*I was in the bathroom at work one day, and I went to unbutton my pants and the button popped off. Boing! My first reaction was 'Man, I gotta lose some weight.' I cinched my belt and went back to my desk and stayed there the rest of the day so nobody would see it.*"

On the T plan's biggest challenge: "*I'm a carb addict, so the first 2 days, I was grumpy. But I found that I wasn't hungry. And after about a week, I saw I was already losing weight, so I was psyched.*"

On his increasing muscle: "*The last 3 weeks, I lost only 2 more pounds, but I was also gaining muscle. My wife told me, 'You have good guns [arms].'*"

On his sex life: "*[Used to be,] you feel like getting it on with your wife, but you're tired and you say, 'Tomorrow.' One Sunday a few weeks ago, my wife and I got it on three times. We hadn't done that since the early years of dating. She'd be mortified if she knew I told you that. We feel like newlyweds again. Our love life is back to when we first started dating, 8 years ago.*"

Bottom line: "*It's definitely changed the way I eat. I eat the right foods and the right amounts, and I don't want to go back to my old bad habits.*"

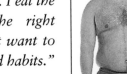

GREG KEMLER, 36, 5' 9"

VITAL STATS		BEFORE T PLAN	AFTER T PLAN
	WEIGHT	195 lb	181 lb
	WAIST	40½"	37"
	BENCH PRESS	170 lb	190 lb
	CHINUPS	2	5

approximating those you'd expect to find in normal, healthy younger men). The study concluded that T improved cardiac bloodflow to the tune of some 17 percent, even in men with established coronary artery disease.

🜨 An Italian research team looked at 14 male heart patients who normally experienced chest pain with exercise. The men's symptoms abated when they were dosed with T prior to treadmill endurance tests.

🜨 In a study involving men suspected of having impaired bloodflow to their hearts, researchers treated the 50 subjects with T for 4 to 8 weeks and found clinically significant improvements in their hearts' oxygen supplies.

🜨 Still skeptical? One of the more ambitious research undertakings examined testosterone and overall health in 4,393 men ages 32 to 48. Testosterone was measured in plasma from blood drawn at 8:00 A.M. Concentrations ranged from 53 nanograms per deciliter (ng/dl) to 1,500, with an average of 679. Researchers found a clear, inverse relationship between T levels and cardiac-risk factors: For example, men with 800 ng/dl of T were 72 percent less likely to have had a heart attack than those with 400 ng/dl. Men with 600 ng/dl were 31 percent less likely to have high diastolic blood pressure than men with 400 ng/dl.

It's worth noting that men with 800 ng/dl were also 8 percent less likely to have three or more colds per year and 75 percent less likely to be obese than those with 400 ng/dl.

Now let's move on to some of the other "incidental" benefits you may enjoy as a result of higher T levels.

KEEPING ALZHEIMER'S IN CHECK

The tragic and debilitating condition known as Alzheimer's disease is marked by the appearance in the brain of so-called senile plaques. These consist of clumps of protein known as beta-amyloid peptides. In a study by researchers at the Rockefeller University and the Weill Medical College of Cornell University in New York City that was funded in part by the U.S. Public Health Service, higher T levels seemed to inhibit the formation of these plaques or break them into harmless fragments. Now, it so happens the researchers did their work on rodents, so we can't necessarily draw hard-and-fast conclusions about what would occur in men. Still, the results were dramatic: The harmful agents were reduced by up to 45 percent. What's more, these findings tally with previous epidemiological studies wherein estrogen, the female rough equivalent of testosterone, was shown to protect postmenopausal women in similar fashion.

BACK TO THAT MORNING ERECTION . . .

There are reams of data on this, but we'll focus on just the latest stuff. We already mentioned a study of AndroGel wherein the 227 subjects experienced clinically important improvements in both sex drive and function.

This is not surprising considering data that show a marked *loss* of sexual function in the presence of declining levels of T. For example, a study at the University of Massachusetts Medical School involving 1,522 men ages 40 to 70 found that protein-deficient diets led to decreased T activity, which in turn caused declines in sexual performance.

In a second study of men with underactive testes, twice-daily T dosing for 8 weeks increased sexual function, as measured by the appearance of spontaneous nocturnal erections. Yes, one could argue that the T merely caused the men to have racy dreams, hence the hard-ons. Even if that's true, it still points to a stepped-up state of overall arousal—more sexy thoughts, a heightened state of sexual "alert"—which can't be all bad.

Another interesting study links exercise, T levels, and sex. Researchers put 78 previously sedentary men on a 9-month exercise regimen. Analysis of the subjects' diary entries revealed that participants enjoyed more frequent sexual activity, more reliable sexual function, and more satisfying orgasms. The researchers theorized that apart from simply and directly improving the men's overall physical condition—thus enhancing their fitness for sex—the exercise may also have boosted T levels, helping them achieve and maintain erections.

And while it's only indirectly relevant to the goals of this book, let's not forget the evidence that regular sex itself just may help keep you alive longer. University of Bristol researchers studied 918 men in the Welsh town of Caerphilly and found that, over a decade, those who had two or more orgasms a week (during sex) were half as likely to have had a heart attack or stroke. Normally, we might be inclined to quibble with such a study on the grounds that it overlooked an obvious flaw: like, maybe the guys who had all those orgasms were in better health to begin with, in which case they were probably more attractive, in which case they had an easier time finding women willing to sleep with them. In other words, we've got a chicken-or-the-egg dilemma on our hands.

Still, it's fun to contemplate the implications of all these studies: More testosterone equals more sex equals more years. And of course, more years of sex.

Wouldn't it be glorious if all this just happened on its own? Sorry, guy. Getting your T to perk up isn't a simple matter of grabbing a barbell and doing a few curls now and then. You need to know what to do to maximize your performance, and you have to avoid getting in your own way. We'll cover all that.

The way you eat is also going to have a lot to say about the success of your Testosterone Advantage Plan. In fact, it has more of an overall impact than the weight-training program. The hows and whys await you.

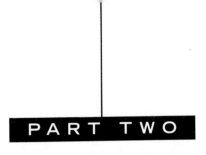

PART TWO

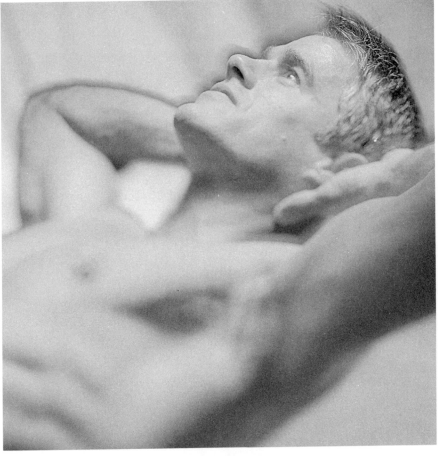

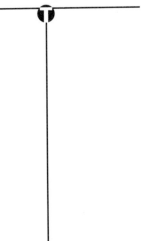

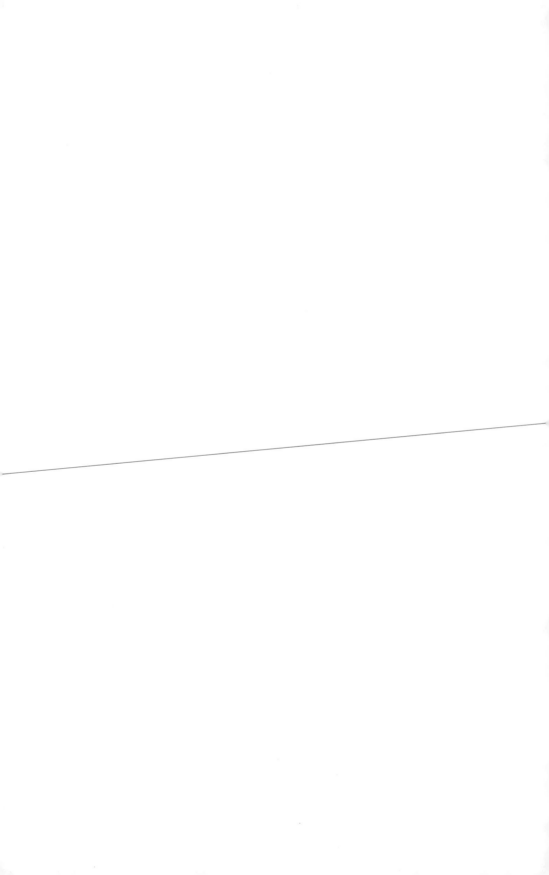

The
Men's Health T

*S*o far, we've been shooting fish in a barrel, blowing holes in the Food Guide Pyramid and aerobics-first exercise plans. You may be thinking, "It's easy to point fingers. But what do *you* have to offer?"

**We hereby present our new paradigm:
the *Men's Health* T.**

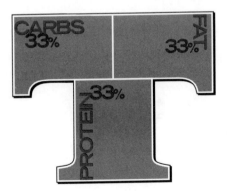

The base of the T is protein, 2 grams for every kilogram (2.2 pounds) of body weight. This is the maximum amount of protein that a weight-lifting man can use to build muscle. The USDA's pyramid scheme is based on minimums—just 0.8 gram of protein per kilogram of body weight—because that's what a sedentary person needs to keep his body from cannibalizing its muscle tissue for energy and organ maintenance.

When you want to build muscle, you need to think about maximums. You want to add as much muscle to your body as possible because that will speed up your metabolism and lead the assault on your body's fat. And protein itself will speed up your metabolism and slow down your appetite. Of the three macronutrients—fat, carbohydrate, protein—it's the one that makes you feel fullest fastest. In addition, your body uses more energy to process protein than it does to process the other two. In other words, just by eating protein, you burn more calories than you would by eating carbs or fat.

Your protein intake will remain constant for as long as you stay on the T diet. But protein as a percentage of the total calories in your diet will increase or decrease depending on your goals, and the proportions of your *Men's Health* T will change to reflect this. For example, if you're trying to lose flab, you'll be eating fewer total calories without changing your protein intake. So you'll base your diet plan on the standard T shown on page 57, with a ratio of one-third protein, one-third fat, and one-third carbohydrate.

If you're trying to bulk up, the arms of your T will get wider as you add calories. The protein base of your T will get shorter since it will now be a smaller percentage of your total calories, leaving you with about 20 percent protein, 40 percent fat, and 40 percent carbs.

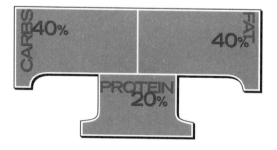

If you're trying to maintain your weight while adding muscle and losing fat, the base of the T will get proportionally longer, representing 25 percent protein, with the remaining 75 percent split evenly between fat and carbs.

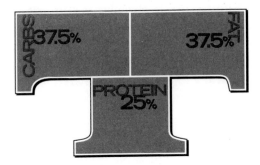

We'll show you, in chapter 9, exactly how to adjust your total calories to fit your particular needs: fat loss, muscle gain, or weight maintenance.

The two arms of the T are likely its most controversial feature. Traditionally, carbohydrate and fat have been kept separate and unequal in dietary recommendations. Carbs get the big, wide space at the base of the Food Guide Pyramid, while fat occupies that little prison cell at the top. And as we've shown, despite research that is clearly rehabilitating fat's role in the diet, it has remained largely stigmatized in the American consciousness. Why? The answer probably has to do with the fact that, as our co-author Dr. Volek explains, "people like simplicity. It's very easy to buy into the concept that if you eat fat, you will get fat. Its not so easy to believe that if you eat fat, you will lose fat."

In any case, here's why we've given carbs and fat equality.

🇹 First, and most important for the Testosterone Advantage Plan, fat is crucial in the production of testosterone. Carbohydrate isn't.

🇹 Second, the types of fat we recommend can readily be used for energy, taking away the need for a carbohydrate-heavy diet.

🇹 Third, these fats are good for your heart and, studies show, for your mood and your general sense of well-being.

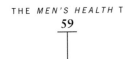

☉ Fourth, of the three macronutrients, fat is the slowest to leave your stomach after a meal. While protein makes you feel full the fastest, fat makes you stay full the longest. That means it takes longer for you to feel hungry again. In fact, most of the guys who used the T diet in our pilot study reported that not only did they not get hungry between meals, they weren't all that hungry at chow time, either.

This raises the question: Why eat carbohydrate at all? If you have protein to build muscle and fat to provide energy, why not just do the full-on Atkins thing?

The short answer is that carbohydrate contains vitamins, minerals, and other vital nutrients that you don't get from other foods and can't get in pill form. So we've included plenty of fruits and vegetables and some whole grains in our T diet. We'll also show you the importance of postexercise carbs when you're trying to build muscle.

Read on, and we'll take a look at the specifics.

CHAPTER
6

The Meat/Muscle Connection

*P*rotein is one of the great battlegrounds in nutrition science today. On the one hand, the nutritional establishment recommends 0.8 gram of protein per kilogram of body weight per day. If you're 180 pounds, that means about 65 grams of protein a day. That's not much. A breakfast of steak and eggs about covers it.

On the other hand, you have books like *Protein Power*, *The Zone*, and *Dr. Atkins' New Diet Revolution* calling for much higher levels.

As is so often the case amid the fog of war—we're talking battlefields here, remember?—both sides are partly right and partly wrong. And none of these recommendations fits a man who's lifting weights with the intention of adding muscle and burning fat. But before we get into that—and show you why the T diet will work better for you than any of the alternatives—let's take a closer look at what protein is and what it does.

THE MULTITASKING MACRONUTRIENT

Protein is found in your body in several different forms.

STRUCTURE. Protein forms the framework of all tissues—muscles,

(continued on page 64)

Bye to Booze

You could see the eyes roll, hear the groans, smell 30 volunteers break out in a cold sweat. The question was simple: "Can we drink while we're on the Testosterone Advantage Plan?" Our answer was even simpler: "No."

We don't know how many guys opted out of our pilot program because of the no-beer dictum, but we could certainly feel the enthusiasm in the room deflate.

It's not that we have anything against alcohol. We just couldn't launch guys on a muscle-building, fat-burning diet-and-workout plan without telling them the truth: Muscle and alcohol go together like Samson and the Flowbee.

Several groups of researchers have looked at how alcohol affects body composition, and the results are fairly consistent in one area: People who drink the most alcohol have the highest waist-to-hip ratios. That is, their waistlines are larger in relation to their hips than those of teetotalers.

This happens for two reasons. First, alcohol causes your body to store fat in your midsection. Second, according to a 1993 study published in *Metabolism*, it also seems to have a wasting effect on thigh and gluteal muscles.

Bigger waist, smaller muscles—we have to think that's the opposite of what you wanted when you bought this book.

This booze-is-bad message is probably confusing, considering all the attention that's been focused on the life-prolonging, heart-protecting benefits of moderate drinking. Not to mention the fact that alcohol increases exponentially your chances of getting lucky on any given Saturday night.

Further complicating this discussion is the fact that alcohol doesn't necessarily make you fatter overall. An intriguing editorial that appeared in a 2000 issue of the *American Journal of Gastroenterology* explained the implications of research regarding the effects of alcohol on body composition. One particular study discussed, which was also presented for the first time in the same issue of the journal, showed that chronic, heavy-duty drinkers were leaner than moderate drinkers. Even though they consumed more total calories, they actually weighed the same as moderate drinkers and had less total fat.

Researchers aren't exactly sure why this was the case. They theorize that alcohol may have a thermogenic effect—that is, it prompts your body to burn more calories than the booze itself contains. So if you down a 900-calorie six-pack, you might expend even more calories getting rid of it.

All of this would appear to give you a license to swill, except for what we've already mentioned: Alcohol deposits fat in your midsection and wastes muscle you already have. Despite having less overall fat, the barflies talked about in the *American Journal of Gastroenterology* still had higher waist-to-hip ratios than moderate drinkers. So they had less total fat, but more in their midsections. Plus, they had scrawnier legs and butts, due to muscle wasting. This left them with your typical big ol' overhanging brew guts, which are bad not only because they're unattractive but also because they're associated with alcoholic liver disease and increased risk for heart disease.

It's possible that the fat-storing, muscle-wasting mechanism could be the work of the stress hormone cortisol. A 2000 study in the *Journal of Applied Physiology* looked at the effects of alcohol on hormones following an intense weight workout. It found that cortisol rose 61 percent higher when alcohol followed weight lifting. Since this was a small study—just nine men—that figure isn't considered statistically significant. However, the study authors speculated that this increased cortisol could, over time, lead to muscle breakdown and hinder the normal increases in strength and muscle mass that you expect from weight training.

So just like those guys who came to hear us pitch our pilot program, you have to ask yourself which is more important to you: drinking suds or becoming a stud.

organs, bones, skin, and connective tissues such as tendons and cartilage.

ENZYMES. These specialized proteins help your body with such vital functions as digestion and energy generation.

HORMONES. Some hormones, such as insulin, are proteins. Hormones act as messengers, telling your body when to be pumped up or stressed out, when to use food for energy and when to store it as fat, when to be a horn-dog and when to go monastic.

TRANSPORTERS. The protein hemoglobin shuttles oxygen through the blood to your muscles and organs, keeping them alive.

MUSCLE CONTRACTORS. Your muscles work by contracting, and contractions are facilitated by little protein filaments called actin and myosin. The bigger and stronger you get, the more actin and myosin you add to your muscles.

ANTIBODIES. These, too, are proteins, and when your body is attacked by viruses and bacteria, they swing into action, protecting you from illness.

Given all that, you'd think that the more protein you gave your body, the more it would use to supply you with stronger antibodies and bigger muscles and more efficient hormones. Not so. Any nutritionist will tell you that if you're sedentary and you go beyond the minimal amount the USDA recommends, you'll just burn off the excess as energy.

See, much as we try to sidestep giving the USDA credit for anything, it so happens that their protein recommendation isn't a made-up number. It's based on your body's nitrogen balance—how much of the element is going into you in the form of nitrogen-rich food and how much is coming out of you in the form of various stuff that comes out of you. Protein is approximately 16 percent nitrogen, so measuring the amount of nitrogen going in and coming out helps reveal whether your body is using the protein or shuttling it into the municipal sewer system.

When intake exceeds excretion, you are said to be in positive nitrogen balance. Because this generally indicates that protein is being retained by your body, we can assume that protein is also being used to build muscle. When the reverse situation develops—that is, when excretion exceeds intake—it means that protein is being degraded within your body at a greater rate than that at which it's being replaced. It also means that your body is breaking down its own protein because it's not getting enough from your diet. This is negative nitrogen balance, and it's a state you don't want to be in if you're serious about making the most of your body. When does it happen? At what level of protein intake and outgo? It's hard for us to give you a set figure because there are so many variables involved, including body type, weight, and caloric intake.

We can tell you that if you don't exercise much and you aren't trying to lose fat, it doesn't take a whole lot of protein to keep you in positive nitrogen balance. But if you *are* trying to lose fat, protein is your best friend. Here's why.

PROTEIN PREVENTS YOU FROM OVEREATING

Numerous studies tell us that if meals are based on protein, you feel full faster and automatically eat less; the effect is known as satiety. Worth noting is a particularly interesting study, published in 1999 in the *European Journal of Clinical Nutrition*. On four separate occasions, 16 guys were fed one of four types of shakes: either 60 percent protein, 60 percent carbohydrate, 60 percent fat, or a mixture with equal amounts of all three macronutrients. (In each of the first three shakes, the other two macronutrients made up the remaining 40 percent.) Two hours later, the guys were led to a lunch spread and invited to chow down. The ones who had drunk the high-protein and mixed-nutrient shakes ate the least for lunch.

Exactly how a high-protein diet makes you feel full is something of a mystery, but as your suddenly skinny ex-wife may have discovered, a person who sticks with a protein-packed diet can get trimmer. Nutritionists scoff at such a diet, saying much of the loss is just water. And even when it's not, they say, it isn't the high protein content that makes the diet work. It's the fact that overall calories are lower.

To which we say, "Your point being . . . ?" What was all that extra fluid doing in your body in the first place, other than making you look like John Goodman? Besides, when you're on a high-protein diet, you can drink gallons of water a day and not gain back those 5 pounds of "water weight" you lost initially. We'll explain why later in this chapter.

As for the nutritionists' second point, that it's the reduction in calories, not the protein content, that makes the diet work for you . . . Look, let's face it, we're guys. We tend to like protein in our diets. So if getting to eat more protein helps cushion the blow of having to eat less food overall, that's good enough for us. Anything that helps us stick with positive eating habits is a plus. We already noted that one of the least-talked-about factors in fitness is *compliance*. No matter how nutritionally sound a given eating or workout plan may be, if it's impossible to stick with, who benefits? A similar dilemma once universally faced owners of British roadsters: The cars looked great in the garage but were useful only for driving to the repair shop and back. They just weren't serviceable for real life. So it is with some of these bizarre diets you can't stay on.

If it's easier for us to stay faithful to a low-calorie diet because it's high in protein, what's the problem?

PROTEIN SPEEDS METABOLISM

You've heard the phrase *It takes money to make money*. (We use it all the time to explain to our wives why we have none.) It also takes energy to make energy. Food contains energy in the form of chemical bonds, but your body cannot use energy in that form. It first has to break down the food to extract the energy from the chemical bonds, a process that itself *requires* energy. In other words, your body has to burn a few calories in order to get the energy from the food you eat.

It takes far more energy to break down protein than to digest other nutrients—2½ times more than to break down carbohydrate, according to the generally accepted formula. This, despite the fact that a gram of protein and a gram of carbohydrate each can provide, on average, about 4 calories of energy. So when you supply your body with protein fuel, at least in digestive terms, you're getting more bang for the buck.

Normally, about 10 percent of the total calories you burn in a day are spent digesting the food you eat. That is called the thermic effect of feeding. (Memorize that phrase. It may come in handy someday when Regis Philbin calls.) When you increase your protein intake—from the USDA recommendation to the T-diet prescription, for example—your body uses more calories to break down that additional protein.

This is one of the reasons why we say the Testosterone Advantage Plan produces *metabolic* weight control: With greater consumption of protein, your body automatically burns more calories throughout the day. And it burns still more when you combine the protein and the T workouts to help you build more metabolically active muscle mass (that is, tissue that keeps your body's calorie-burning function humming happily along).

Say you eat 2,500 calories a day on a standard-issue "healthy" diet of about 15 percent protein, 25 percent fat, and 60 percent carbohydrate. Let's do some math, using the generally accepted figures for the thermic effects of protein (20 percent, or .2, of calories consumed), fat (2 percent, or .02), and carbs (8 percent, or .08).

Here's how many calories you'd burn each day through the thermic effect of feeding alone (all calories in these examples are rounded off to the nearest whole number).

PROTEIN $2,500 \times 15\% = 375 \times .2 = 75$

FAT $2,500 \times 25\% = 625 \times .02 = 13$

CARBOHYDRATE $2,500 \times 60\% = 1,500 \times .08 = 120$

The total is 208 thermic calories used.

Now here's what happens when you shift to a diet consisting of one-third (33⅓ percent) protein, one-third fat, and one-third carbs.

PROTEIN $2,500 \times 33\frac{1}{3}\% = 833 \text{ calories} \times .2 = 167$

FAT $2,500 \times 33\frac{1}{3}\% = 833 \text{ calories} \times .02 = 17$

CARBOHYDRATE $2,500 \times 33\frac{1}{3}\% = 833 \times .08 = 67$

The new total is 251, or an increase of 43 calories per day. Over a year, that's 15,695 calories, or almost 4½ pounds' worth. These results are even more startling in percentage terms: You have upped your metabolic calorie burning by a fast 20.75 percent—by doing nothing more energetic than adjusting the relative quantities of the macronutrients you eat!

At this point, we hope you're wondering the same thing we often wonder: If a higher-protein diet is so damn good for your waistline, why

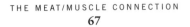

does the mainstream nutritional establishment have such a negative attitude toward protein? How come, when you talk to a dietitian, you walk away thinking that protein will make your kidneys fall out?

Some prominent researchers have also wondered this and set out to find answers.

MAYBE JOCKS AREN'T SO DUMB AFTER ALL

Meet one of the most widely quoted exercise scientists alive: Peter W. R. Lemon, Ph.D., professor and Weider chair of exercise nutrition at the University of Western Ontario. Lemon's studies on the protein requirements for muscle-building athletes are the basis for most recommendations today, including those in this book.

As he recalls in a 1996 paper published in *Nutrition Reviews*, Lemon first started researching protein as a grad student around 1975 because he was intrigued by the huge split between research and practice. Researchers had concluded earlier in the century that the protein needs of athletes were actually very small, and yet athletes were consuming high-protein diets.

Could it be that athletes, in general, and muscleheads, in particular, knew something that all the esteemed scientists in exercise nutrition had missed? By 1992, Lemon and others had concluded that men lifting heavy weights needed 1.7 to 1.8 grams of protein per kilogram of body weight per day, or more than twice the amount recommended by the USDA. As we stated in the previous chapter, we round those numbers up a bit for our T diet, to 2 grams per kilogram per day. Most bodybuilders notch them up even higher, to about 2.2 grams per kilogram. Anything above that is almost certainly superfluous from a bodybuilding standpoint because there's an upper limit to what the body can process. Studies peg this limit at upward of 2.4 grams per kilogram per day.

WILL INCREASED PROTEIN REALLY REQUIRE YOU TO GET ON AN ORGAN-TRANSPLANT WAITING LIST?

The controversy over protein intake didn't end with the debate about how much protein you should eat. Nutritionists brought up a laundry list of supposed protein-related health risks. We'll take each in turn.

KIDNEY DAMAGE. Protein does require your kidneys to work harder than they do when you're eating a diet loaded with carbs and fat. But making them *work* is not the same as making them *sick*. Look at it this way: When you think hard, you make your brain work hard. Is that bad for you? Not at all. In fact, research increasingly suggests that intense mental activity helps ward off such conditions as Alzheimer's disease.

If protein made kidneys fail, there would be millions of bodybuilders, powerlifters, football players, and wrestlers on dialysis. There aren't. Or as Lemon put it, "Potential kidney problems have been extrapolated from studies on individuals with impaired kidney function." In other words, if there's something wrong with your kidneys to start with, they may have trouble handling the extra load. That's no different from what happens in the case of almost any other disability. How is that protein's fault?

Everyone does seem to agree that protein leads to some fluid loss. Combine a higher-protein diet with vigorous exercise, and you're going to have a fair amount of pissing and sweating. The reason? Actually there are two. First, a high-protein, low-carbohydrate diet may somewhat deplete your glycogen stores, which provide you with the energy you need to tap into when you work out. For every stored glycogen molecule, you also store 2 to 3 grams of water. When the glycogen is broken down for energy, this water is released. The second reason is that your kidneys pull more water from your stores to break down the extra protein.

Okay, now pay close attention because we're about to impart a brilliant piece of physiological wisdom.

Drink some extra water.

How much, you ask? See "The Wet Look" on page 72.

Problem solved.

BONE LOSS. One 1979 study suggested that a high-protein diet causes your body to lose calcium through urination, leading to weaker bones. But a 1985 study showed that is more of a problem with *purified* proteins, such as those in meal-replacement supplements like MET-Rx or Myoplex.

The natural, unpurified protein in actual food has a high phosphorus content, negating the pissed-away-bones effect. It works like this: The mineral phosphorus helps to decrease the amount of calcium that's excreted in your urine and increase the amount that's reabsorbed back into your body.

HEART DISEASE. Another fear is that a higher-protein diet is associated with higher saturated fat intake, leading to increased risk of heart disease. That's a debatable point on many levels. For one thing, bodybuilders who eat mountains of skinless chicken breasts take in a minimal amount of fat. Plus, saturated fat is certainly not an issue on the T diet. That's because most of the fat you'll eat is monounsaturated, and we'll explain in the next chapter why that is actually *good* for your heart.

The biggest fear nutritionists toss out, though, is that higher-protein diets decrease testosterone. Since that allegation, if true, would negate the entire premise of the book you're reading, it bears some special scrutiny.

THE BULL

Protein detractors tend to point to a 1987 study that "proved" that high protein levels lower testosterone. The study involved seven subjects who ate a 44-percent-protein diet for 10 days, then switched over to a 10-percent-protein diet for the next 10 days. Their T levels were measured as 28 percent higher on the lower-protein diet.

A few observations:

The seven subjects in the study had an average body weight of 150 pounds and ate an average of 275 grams of protein a day during the high-protein phase. That's about 4 grams of protein per kilogram of body weight, or twice what our T diet recommends. (The 10-percent-protein diet was 0.9 gram per kilogram of body weight, or just above the USDA recommendation.)

Both diets were low in fat—about 20 percent of total calories. Fat, as you've already heard and as we'll explain in more detail in the next chapter, is the primary building block of T.

Another point worth making is that this study didn't seem to have any real-world context. The only people we know of who follow such high-protein, low-fat diets are serious bodybuilders, who use them as a pure muscle-building tool. And yet, there was no exercise component to the study! The researchers didn't even measure body fat to see if the protein eaters had gotten leaner over the 4 weeks.

The bottom line is, to separate a bodybuilding diet from bodybuilding exercise is to load the body with tons of high-octane fuel without providing a mechanism for burning that fuel off. That's not unlike eating and eating without ever excreting—as you might imagine, you'd be apt to get some pretty weird bodily reactions. Moreover, you'd have to wonder if you'd really learned anything useful from the "experiment."

THE BEEF

Now let's look at a more recent study, published in 2000. Researchers drew blood from 1,552 men—for the math-impaired, that's more than seven—participating in the Massachusetts Male Aging Study. The participants' mean age was 55.

The researchers found that the lower the protein intake, the higher the levels of sex-hormone-binding globulin, a chemical that attaches to T and keeps it from becoming bioavailable. When T isn't bioavailable, your body can't use it to make muscle, maintain sex drive, or do any of the other helpful things we described in chapter 4.

Unfortunately, we can't make sweeping conclusions based on either of the above studies, since they're both somewhat flawed. The first was an intervention study, meaning the researchers took a small group of guys (a really small group of guys), changed their diets, and measured what happened. We can't assume that what happened to those seven men would occur at the same rate among a larger group. The second study was a large cross-section that looked at more than 1,500 men, but the researchers didn't intervene to see if changing the guys' diets would alter their T levels. Without such an intervention, we can't definitely say that the guys' low-protein intakes were the sole cause of their elevated sex-hormone-binding globulin.

We also feel compelled to note that neither study was conducted using

The Wet Look

On a manliness scale from 1 to 10, sweating always earns you high marks. You get a 6 if you sweat lifting weights, an 8 if you sweat lifting weights naked with Miss Oklahoma, and a 10 if you sweat because the tank that you drove to the gym in isn't air-conditioned.

Just realize one thing amid all these visions of a naked Miss Oklahoma: Sweating drains fluid from your body, which is actually about 60 percent water. Your muscles are about 80 percent water. So how do you think your body performs when it's running a pint low on the H_2O?

Let's run the numbers: Say you're a strapping 180-pounder. At 60 percent of your body weight, that's 108 pounds of water. When you lose 1 percent of it—a little more than a pound, or 1 pint, of fluid—you start feeling fatigued and irritable (not exactly what Miss Oklahoma was expecting). You have a greater chance of passing out from the heat (a real liability in a tank battle). Your exercise per-

formance suffers, you recover more slowly, and you become more susceptible to colds, flu, and other infections. Not feeling so macho anymore, huh?

On the other hand, real health benefits accrue when you top off your radiator. A study of 47,909 men sponsored by Harvard University found that for every 8 ounces of fluid you drink in an average day, you lower your risk of bladder cancer by 7 percent. The study also found that a high fluid intake reduces your risk for kidney stones.

We even have a vanity angle here. When you don't drink enough water, ironically, your body retains fluid, making you look tired and puffy and obscuring whatever muscle you have. But when your body gets enough water, it doesn't bother holding on to any extra, and you find that you can actually see your biceps—not to mention your cheekbones.

Hydration takes on even greater importance when you start the Testosterone Advantage Plan. First off, the higher protein intake causes you to lose a few pounds of water almost immediately. Second, the workouts make you sweat like a gladiator if you do them right. So the day you start this program is the day you have to get serious about pouring more water down your throat.

All Along the Water Tower

How much fluid do you need? It depends. The amount of perspiration you produce depends on a few factors, including genetics. (Here's a fun fact: The size of your pores, which is genetically determined, helps determine how much you sweat.) Another determinant is the shape you're in. Sweating is your body's way of controlling its temperature, and a well-trained body is better at this than a poorly conditioned one.

There are two pretty easy ways to determine if you're drinking too little or too much, and they both involve urine. You can tell that you're running low if your urine is dark and has a strong odor. Another tip-off is that you don't go very often, and when you do, you don't exactly hose down the porcelain.

Clear and odorless whiz means you're carrying a full load. But if you're unloading so much clear and odorless urine that you have to interrupt your work every 15 minutes, you can safely guess you're overdoing it.

A slightly more scientific way to calculate fluid loss is to weigh yourself immediately before and after exercise (a digital scale is helpful). For this one test only, don't drink any fluid during your workout. The difference between your pre- and post-workout weights is the amount of fluid you lose in a typical workout. A pound of body weight equals 16 ounces of water. So if you lose 3 pounds, you know you need to take in 48 ounces of fluid.

Most guys need 5 to 6 pints—80 to 96 ounces—of fluid per day. And that's on the days they don't exercise. On workout days, they need an additional 2 to 3 pints. That means most guys do fine with about a gallon of fluid on the days they exercise.

The easiest way to fulfill your fluid requirement is simply to drink a quart (32-ounce) bottle of water three times a day. Don't bother with those chichi wimp waters with names like Crystal Cool Aspen Spring and Le Scheme de Marketeurs. They send the manly meter plunging down to −3. Just get some fresh-squeezed tap water, chug it, and wipe your mouth on your sleeve. Then fill the bottle up a fourth time, and offer Miss Oklahoma a swig. After all, you don't want her to become fatigued and irritable, either.

a group of guys actively lifting weights. Therefore, why not take a look at what protein can do for your body when you throw some dumbbells into the mix?

HOW MEAT MAKES MUSCLE

More protein doesn't automatically translate to more muscle, but the right amount of protein, combined with the right type of exercise, can increase muscle dramatically. This process works two ways: by building new muscle (anabolism) and by preventing muscle breakdown (catabolism).

ANABOLISM. The creation of new muscle, paradoxically, starts with muscle damage. Lifting and lowering heavy objects creates microscopic tears in muscle cells.

(Timeout for a quick pop quiz: Which action creates more such tears: lifting the weight or lowering the weight? Lifting it, of course. That's why it's called *weight lifting*, right? Wrong. Lowering the weight actually does more of this damage.)

Like a good earthquake, this provides an opportunity to make the original structure stronger, which your body does by adding protein to the muscle cells. A single workout can create a muscle-building "anabolic environment" in the targeted cells that lasts 24 to 48 hours—even longer, if you have a significant amount of muscle cell damage. By "anabolic environment" we're referring to the tears that require repairing as well as to the testosterone spike and the step-up in protein synthesis (the use of protein to help make new muscle fibers) that also occur after a workout. These three anabolic components work together to make you stronger than ever.

Lift weights three times a week in a progressive program like the one in this book, and your body stays in a muscle-building mode pretty much all day, every day.

CATABOLISM. There's more to building muscle than just slapping new protein on the old. You have to prevent the old from breaking down too far before the reinforcements arrive. Proper nutrition limits that breakdown.

Here's what happens: During a hard workout, your body runs short of its preferred fuel, glycogen, and starts pulling protein out of your muscles to use for energy. (By the way, this is a much bigger issue for aerobic athletes than for weight lifters, but it happens to everyone who trains hard.) If you keep your body constantly supplied with high-quality dietary protein, you minimize this cannibalistic breakdown.

Maximize both sides of the equation—good, muscle-challenging workouts and effective, muscle-sparing meals—and you'll get the best body possible.

THE THREE AMINOS

Protein is made of amino acids. Some are called essential amino acids, meaning your body can't produce them and must get them from your food. The best protein sources contain all nine of the essential amino acids in relatively the same amounts that your body requires. The next best contain all of the essential aminos, but a few of the values fall below your body's needs. The worst proteins are either missing an amino altogether or provide low values of most or all of the essential aminos.

Here's a quick rundown of the three tiers of amino acids.

BEST: Dairy products (especially cottage cheese), eggs, beef, pork, poultry, fish, oats, nuts, and soy protein

NEXT BEST: Beans, seeds, and cornmeal

WORST: White or wheat bread, peas, rice, potatoes, pasta, and gelatin

At this point, you may wonder why vegetarians don't collapse into gelatinous heaps from eating foods missing essential aminos. That's because your body can combine incomplete proteins to make complete ones. The only problem with this strategy is that relying on incomplete proteins can lead to incomplete muscle development. We don't mean that the muscles themselves will be incomplete—your vegan friend isn't missing half a biceps. He just won't grow as much muscle as we meat eaters do, when all else is equal.

An interesting 1999 study compared the muscle-building effects of two different diets on 19 overweight, sedentary men ages 51 to 69. Nine of the men ate a diet in which half the protein came from meat and other animal sources—a typical Western diet. The other 10 ate a vegetarian diet that included dairy and eggs (but, obviously, no meat). Both groups were put on the same weight-lifting program.

Look at the results that the study found after 12 weeks.

	MEAT-EATERS	VEGETARIANS
Muscle	Gained 3.74 lb	Lost 1.76 lb
Fat	Lost 2.86 lb	Gained 0.22 lb

A Dutch study published in 1992 looked at changes in T levels on these two diets. A group of young male endurance athletes ate and trained on each diet for 6 weeks. (Half started on the meat-rich diet, half on the vegetarian diet; then they switched.) Total testosterone declined 35 percent when the athletes used the vegetarian diet. Unfortunately, the researchers didn't record changes in fat and muscle mass from one diet to the other.

So one study shows that meat equals muscle, and another study shows that meat equals testosterone. The message seems clear: Pack the occasional slab of animal flesh in your lunchbox.

PUMPING THE NUMBERS

It stands to reason that a guy who's exercising needs more protein than a guy who isn't, and indeed, research has shown this to be true. The big challenge is figuring out how much the exerciser needs and at what point protein consumption reaches overkill.

As we said earlier in this chapter, the most reliable research shows that strength and power athletes need 1.7 to 1.8 grams of daily protein per kilogram of body weight to build and repair muscle. We also noted that 2.4 grams per kilogram was overkill.

In composing our T diet, we decided to use a number in between those two—2 grams per kilogram, or 164 grams of protein a day for a 180-pound guy. Even if some of it is overkill for the muscle-building side, we want you to have the extra protein for the benefits on the metabolic side.

And, of course, we want to leave room in your diet for the two arms of the T: fats and carbohydrate. Read on. . . .

CHAPTER

7

The
Manly Fats

*T*hroughout the "diet wars," amid the countless revisions and rethinkings and debates and controversies over what people should or shouldn't eat, one notion has remained pretty much constant and unchallenged:

Fat makes you fat.

First of all, it sounds intuitive, commonsensical. The fat on your food looks like the fat on your body. And let's be clear on this: There's a lot of fat in food besides the stuff you can actually see. But the fat you *can* see? Well, visible fat on food has that same squishiness, that same formlessness, that same unappealing quality as the fat on your waist. So the translation between diet and waistline seems to make sense.

Scientifically, meanwhile, the rationale for why fat would make you fat reduces to simple math. A gram of fat contains 9 calories, on average. That's more than twice the calories of a gram of protein or carbohydrate. Plus, fat has the lowest thermic effect of the three macronutrients. It takes the least amount of energy to digest and process in your body.

In other words, fat is pretty much designed for quick and easy storage. Quick and easy and ugly storage.

Furthermore, fat has been linked to heart disease, stroke, obesity, and just about every other plague of modern life, including the shrinking ozone layer. (We're not joking. Flatulent cattle are said to release enough methane to damage the ozone. The more fatty beef we want to eat, the more farting cattle we breed.)

So why the hell are we making fat an equal partner with carbohydrates in this diet? A fair question.

In the previous chapter, we showed that building muscle is a two-part process. The first part is adding protein to muscle, and the second is preventing preexisting muscle protein from being used for energy during and after weight lifting. Fat seems to play a role in the latter, preventive stage.

The evidence supporting fat's muscle-sustaining effects goes back to 1989, when a small but interesting Canadian study appeared in the *American Journal of Clinical Nutrition*. In that study, six male subjects were put on either a high-carbohydrate diet, in which the ratio of carbs to fat was 2:1, or a high-fat diet, in which the ratio was 1:1.

The researchers found that nitrogen retention was higher on the high-fat diet, the one with the 1:1 ratio of carbs to fat. Since in this context the higher the nitrogen levels, the lower the muscle loss, the researchers believed that muscle protein was being spared by the higher-fat diet because fatty acids, instead of carbs, were being used for energy.

Now, in some respects that Canadian study is not directly relevant to the Testosterone Advantage Plan. Unlike the eating plans we're going to give you, the diets tested were low in protein. And the subjects in the study weren't exercising. And, hey, there were only six guys. Still, the results were illuminating. Up until that time, it was assumed—and research had seemed to prove—that carbohydrates had a bigger role in preventing protein breakdown. Fat's role in the muscle-building process had been overlooked.

A more recent study, published in 2001 in the *American Journal of Clinical Nutrition*, tackled the problem from a different direction: It tried to determine what happens when you cut fat calories without cutting total calories. The results indicated that merely cutting the fat in your diet does not, in and of itself, produce loss of body fat. Nor, in the study, did reducing fat intake lead to any significant reductions in factors linked to heart-disease risk. In fact, the levels of one such risk factor—triglycerides in the blood—actually increased on the low-fat diet.

What's more, when the same study cut overall calories in the diet while maintaining a typical American fat intake of 35 percent of calories from fat, the 11 men in the study did reduce their body fat. Logically, this suggests that what's important is the number of calories you take in, all told. For even if a relatively large percentage of those calories comes from fat, you're still going to lose some flab as long as your total caloric intake drops.

What happens when you add exercise to this mix? According to a study by our co-author Dr. Volek, the benefits for men are multiplied—even when fat intake is raised to truly eyebrow-raising proportions. Dr. Volek put 12 normal-weight men who were regular exercisers on a reduced-calorie, high-fat, low-carbohydrate diet and told them to continue their usual exercise regimens for 6 weeks. The subjects actually lost body fat while increasing muscle mass.

And just how high was the high-fat content? Try 70 percent. (Somewhere, an American Heart Association spokesperson is clutching his chest.)

So clearly, the role of fat in your diet is undergoing a major revision.

CHOLESTEROL: THE FULL STORY

Just as nutritionists who focused on lowering fat as the best way to help people control weight actually oversimplified the issue, doctors who focused on "lowering cholesterol" as the best way to fight off heart disease were similarly skimming the surface.

Cholesterol is a waxy substance that's manufactured in your liver and small intestine and found virtually everywhere in your body. (Amaze your friends with this completely trivial fact: Your body weight is about 0.2 percent cholesterol.) Its chemical structure is similar to that of

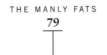

steroids—not surprising when you consider that it's a building block of testosterone and also serves as a chemical ancestor of other hormones that, for better or worse, have major effects on your muscles: progesterone, estrogen, and cortisol.

Cholesterol is carried through your bloodstream by molecules called lipoproteins. There are two main types: low-density lipoproteins (LDL), which carry cholesterol to various tissues, and high-density lipoproteins (HDL), which carry cholesterol back to the liver for removal from your body.

The two have a yin-yang relationship. LDL, the lipoprotein found in the greater concentrations in the blood, creates problems because as it transports the cholesterol to your organs, its lower density allows some of the cholesterol to stick to blood-vessel walls and eventually block them. When the vessels become blocked and bloodflow to your heart stops, your heart itself stops, too. Experts on all sides of the nutrition debate seem to agree that this is not a good thing.

HDL saves your heart by pulling excess cholesterol out of the places where it can work its mischief and returning it to the liver. Thanks to its high density, HDL is able to transport cholesterol without permitting it to stick to artery walls.

The Framingham Heart Study, an ongoing study of over 5,000 people spanning 5 decades, found that a low level of HDL indicates an increased risk for heart disease, regardless of total cholesterol level. A level below 40 milligrams per deciliter is considered dangerous. On the other hand, an HDL level above 60 is considered protective against heart disease.

Thus, elevating LDL is a bad idea, while elevating HDL is great for you. So knowing your total cholesterol level is meaningless if you don't also know your ratio of LDL to HDL.

One other type of blood fat worth mentioning again here is triglycerides. This is the storage form of fat, and elevated levels in the blood are associated with increased risk of heart disease and clogging of the arteries (though the exact physiological mechanism of its evildoing is unknown). A large-scale study in Münster, Germany, found that a high triglycerides level can lead to heart disease regardless of cholesterol level.

So keep three things in mind as you read the next section:

"IT'S EASIER TO GET UP"

Perhaps more than any other participant, Mike Hoye lauded the T plan for boosting his energy—though he sure didn't mind dropping a few waist sizes, either.

On his results: *"The biggest accomplishment was losing substantial inches off my belt, to fit right into those pants you haven't fit into in a while. My best physical attribute now is probably my abs. If I stay on it, I think, I could get a six-pack."*

On the T plan itself: *"I do some martial arts, but I never did weight training. This is a great way to get into a weight program and the nutrition side at the same time. Once I got into the routine of packing lunch the night before, it became easy. I worked out at 6:00 A.M., got to work by 7:30."*

On his stepped-up productivity: *"Overall, I noticed more energy and a sustained level of it. It's easier to get up in the morning. Through the course of a workday, I'm more aggressive toward my work, with a sharper attention span. I'm more effective at setting goals at the beginning of the week and checking them off faster. Not only do I finish my to-do list but I find myself adding more. In the past, I would always have stuff left to carry over into next week."*

Bottom line: *"After 12 hours of work, I still have energy to get down on the floor and roll around with the kids. I'm squeezing more out of every day."*

MIKE HOYE, 35, 6' 3"

VITAL STATS		BEFORE T PLAN	AFTER T PLAN
	WEIGHT	228 lb	212 lb
	WAIST	40"	36"
	CHINUPS	3	7

Lower LDL is good.
Higher HDL is good.
Lower triglycerides are good.

The biggest dangers to your heart arise when you lower your HDL levels or increase your triglyceride level. And the biggest favor you can do for your heart is to raise HDL and lower triglycerides. For a quick reference to exactly how much of each is desirable, take a look at this cheat sheet. Measurements are in milligrams per deciliter (mg/dl) of blood.

	DESIRABLE	BORDERLINE	UNDESIRABLE
Total cholesterol (TC)	< 200	200–239	≥ 240
HDL	≥ 60	40–59	< 40
LDL	< 130*	130–159	≥ 160
Triglycerides	< 150	150–199	≥ 200

*If you have heart disease or diabetes, your LDL goal is < 100

Because your body produces cholesterol, there's no need to get any in your diet. Though most men get 300 to 500 milligrams a day from animal foods (milk, eggs, meat, seafood), your body creates between 600 and 1,500 milligrams all on its own. For several decades, the public has been told that cholesterol in food leads to greater cholesterol in the blood. That is true in some cases, but genetics are always at work when it comes to cholesterol metabolism and absorption. So is the body's tendency to self-regulate. When you eat an abundance of dietary cholesterol, your body tends to produce less. Now, we have a feeling that we know what you're thinking here—and you're wrong: You can't keep your cholesterol levels happily low by eating a dinner of, say, five stuffed-crust pizzas with all the fixings. There are limits to what your body can regulate without medication. The process we're describing merely explains how your body works within more-or-less normal limits—meaning limits that are normal *for you*. What we're trying to get across is that a diet that's super-low in cholesterol will not automatically keep you out of the cardiac-care unit if genetics has predisposed you to have an awful lot of that glop circulating in your blood anyway. And—just as important, for our purposes—a diet containing large amounts of cholesterol will not necessarily send your levels soaring out of control.

If your brows just shot up, you've probably fallen prey to a core misunderstanding that took hold some years back when the medical establishment started warning us about the dangers of cholesterol. We were told, "Eat a cholesterol-lowering diet." What we heard—and a lot of doctors heard it right along with us—was "Eat a low-cholesterol diet." Two different things, with two vastly different implications. We have proof of this in the recent destigmatizing of the once lowly egg: Yes, eggs are relatively high in cholesterol, but they're low in saturated fats.

It's saturated fats—not cholesterol per se— that raise LDL cholesterol inside your body.

Saturated fats are found mostly in animal products such as red meat, poultry, and dairy foods, and they're usually solid at room temperature. Limiting your intake of saturated fats is still important—in our plan, we keep it to around 10 percent of total calories.

But unlike traditional cholesterol-lowering strategies, we don't tell you to replace saturated fats with carbohydrate. We want you to replace it with other, healthier types of fat.

LIVE OFF THE FAT OF THE LAND AND SEA

Remember that study we mentioned in which guys lost body fat while on a low-calorie, 35-percent-fat diet? Those study subjects also experienced reductions in their LDL levels, increases in their HDL levels, and reductions in their triglyceride levels. When they switched to the low-calorie, low-fat diet, they still decreased their LDL and triglycerides. But here's an important kicker: The low-fat, low-calorie diet did not raise HDL cholesterol. The higher-fat diet did. So what are we left with?

The paradoxical-sounding but scientifically defensible conclusion that for men, eating more fat may just be better for overall cholesterol levels than eating less fat.

How is this possible, you ask? Saturated fats do raise LDL levels, but, to a lesser degree, they also lower triglycerides and even raise HDL. Furthermore, there are other kinds of dietary fats whose effects on cholesterol levels are overwhelmingly positive. Perhaps the most important of these beneficial fats are **MONOUNSATURATED FATS**. Liquid at room temperature and found mostly in olive and canola oils and in macadamia nuts, monounsaturates yield a far better effect: You get higher HDL and lower triglycerides. Diets that get about 25 percent of their calories from monounsaturated fats and about 40 percent of total calories from fat have been shown to raise HDL by 8 to 22 percent and decrease triglycerides by up to 24 percent without raising LDL. This, by the way, is the classic Mediterranean diet, which we'll discuss later in this chapter.

Another great benefit is available from replacing some of the carbs in your diet with **POLYUNSATURATED FATS**. These are found in abundance in fish as well as in some oils (particularly safflower and sunflower), nuts, and seeds—and like monounsaturates, they're usually liquid at room temperature. Polyunsaturates are further divided into *omega-3 and omega-6 fatty acids*. The fats in fish and fish oil are omega-3's; fats in plants and plant oils are generally omega-6's. A subset of these are *essential fatty acids*. Your body can't produce these important fats—used in cell membranes and the production of substances that help regulate blood pressure and blood clotting—and thus you have to get them from food. One is an omega-6 fat called linoleic acid, found in safflower oil, walnuts, red meats, and poultry. Another is an omega-3 fat called linolenic acid, found in fatty cold-water fish like tuna and salmon as well as in flaxseed oil.

Supplementing your diet with omega-3 fats in the form of fish oil has been shown to lower triglycerides by 63 percent. (The higher the number you start with, the more dramatic the effect.)

One type of polyunsaturated fats that you should avoid is *trans fats*.

These occur in small amounts in natural foods but in great amounts in processed foods like margarine and baked goods. The term *trans* refers to the fact that the fats are *trans*formed from liquid polyunsaturates to solid fats during a chemical process called hydrogenation (hence, trans fats are also known as *partially hydrogenated fats*). At one point, trans fats were considered a healthy alternative to saturated fats. Consumers were advised to switch from butter to margarine, and fast-food restaurants started using trans fats for frying instead of the beef fat they'd been using.

As it turns out, this was a very bad idea, because trans fats lower HDL while raising total cholesterol and LDL. That's why you won't find doughnuts and nachos anywhere in the T diet. We like that stuff as much as you do, but if you want a good body and a longer life, you have to sacrifice something. Everything has its costs. We just think the costs we ask you to pay in dietary restrictions are far lower than what the nutritional establishment has been preaching at you for decades.

The following table provides a quick summary of what happens to blood-lipid levels when you replace carbohydrates in your diet with the different types of fat. The number of arrows in the following table indicates the magnitude of effect a particular class of fat has on lipid levels in the body. A dash indicates no effect.

	TOTAL CHOLESTEROL	LDL	HDL	TRIGLYCERIDES
Saturated fat	↑↑↑	↑↑↑	↑↑	↓↓
Omega-6 poly-unsaturated fat	↓↓	↓↓	↑	↓↓
Omega-3 poly-unsaturated fat	—	—	—	↓↓↓↓
Monounsaturated fat	↓	↓	↑↑	↓↓
Trans-fatty acids	↑↑	↑↑	↓	↓

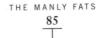

THE T/FAT CONNECTION

Even beyond the advantages of lowering your risk of cardiovascular disease, the greatest benefit of the higher-fat T diet is what it does for your hormones.

Cholesterol is the building block of testosterone, so it makes sense that a meat-eating, cholesterol-consuming diet would yield more of the big T than a vegetarian diet would. And, indeed, that's what a 1985 study found when it looked at a large cross section of omnivores and vegetarians. What was surprising was how significant the difference was: The meat-eaters actually had 36 percent more T than the guys who stuck to rabbit food.

Here are some other interesting differences between the diets of the two groups studied.

	MEAT-EATERS	VEGETARIANS
Fat in overall diet	38%	34%
Daily cholesterol intake	309 mg	197 mg
Daily fiber intake	23 g	37 g

A 1989 study found pretty much the same thing: The meat-eaters ate more fat, more cholesterol, more saturated fat, and less fiber than the vegetarians and had 31 percent more testosterone.

An interesting 1987 study put men on a high-fat diet (about 50 percent of calories from fat) for 2 weeks, then had them switch to a low-fat diet (about 10 percent fat) for 2 weeks. Their free testosterone—the part that's available for use in building muscle—dropped 21 percent on the low-fat diet.

A 1984 study used a less radical switch in daily fat intake, taking men from their customary 40 percent of calories from fat to 25 percent, and studied them over 6 weeks instead of 2. The lower-fat diet decreased testosterone by 15 percent.

Other studies in men—and even studies in women—have found this same effect. Some studies have shown that in the very youngest men (19 years old) there's no difference in testosterone levels between omnivores and vegetarians, but the overall body of research points toward a 40-percent-fat diet as more T-friendly than one with less than 30 percent of calories from fat.

CLUB MEDITERRANEAN

If you had to rank the world's populations in terms of pure hairy-chested manliness, chances are Greeks, Sicilians, and Cypriots would rank at or near the top. So it should be self-evident that an eating plan similar to the classic Mediterranean diet, deriving about 25 to 40 percent of its calories from fat, is optimal for increasing or maintaining your testosterone levels. (If not, sit down and watch *The Godfather*. "Leave the gun. Take the cannoli." See?)

Interest in the Mediterranean diet started in the 1960s, when researchers observed that people in the olive-growing regions lived longer, had less heart disease and fewer heart attacks, and had fewer incidences of some cancers (including prostate cancer, the second-most-deadly cancer for men).

Most of the fat in the Mediterranean diet comes from olive oil, meaning most of it is monounsaturated. The protein comes from fish, eggs, and cheese. The carbohydrate comes from whole grain bread, pasta, and rice as well as from fresh, seasonal fruits and vegetables. The diet has little saturated fat and virtually no refined or sweetened carbohydrate.

Our T diet borrows from the Mediterranean model, although we did make modifications to ensure you get the best results from the complementary T workout plan.

Now let's move on to the last component of our T diet: carbohydrate.

Carbohydrate Revisited

*F*irst off, we'd like to assure you that we aren't really in the anti-carbohydrate camp. We haven't concluded that Americans are getting fatter simply because they're eating less fat and more carbohydrate. We don't believe that beans and grains alone have turned our strapping American youth into a population of porkers.

We do think SnackWell's cookies and similar offerings are crappy products. Not because they're fat-free but because they're nutrient-free. Set a box of SnackWell's (600 calories) next to supersized fries (610 calories) and, in terms of the amount of damage each is capable of producing, they're about equal.

Put bluntly, we believe Americans are getting fatter because they're eating too damn many Bloomin' Onions and watching too damn many episodes of *Survivor*. Indeed, they ought to film *Survivor* in a more appropriate setting—say, a fast-food restaurant: "Who will waddle out alive?"

Our problem with carbohydrate is mostly one of proportion. You don't get fat by eating healthy carbs like fruits, vegetables, whole grains, and beans. In fact, eating more of them is your first line of defense against cancer and other deadly diseases. One specific benefit you should take note of is that whole grains seem to protect against prostate cancer, according to a recent compilation of data from 59 countries.

The thing is, the average guy doesn't find those foods very tasty or satisfying. So we're back to talking about the compliance factor we've already mentioned a couple of times. And you certainly don't want to base your diet on such foods when you're trying to increase testosterone and build muscle.

Let's talk about exactly what carbohydrate does for you—the good, the bad, and the ugly—and how it fits into the T diet.

CLASSIFIED INFORMATION

Part of the confusion surrounding carbohydrate has to do with classification. Up until a few years ago, carbs were usually described as either simple or complex. Simple indicated a carb containing one or two sugar molecules. Examples include sucrose (table sugar), fructose (found, amazingly enough, in fruit), and lactose (dairy products). Complex described the presence of more than two sugar molecules. Those most commonly eaten are starches, such as pasta, rice, bread, and potatoes.

Dietary recommendations based on these two chemical classifications were pretty useless. Many foods containing simple carbs help you stay energized and lean—fruits and low-fat dairy products, for example. The apple that helps keep the doctor away contains simple carbs. But so does table sugar, a food that has no health-promoting nutrients that we know of. Conversely, both the whole grains in oatmeal and the flour in angel food cake were considered complex carbs.

So if someone told you to build your diet around complex carbs instead of simple ones, what did you do? In a universe wherein angel food cake was equivalent to an apple, which did most people choose?

Today, nutritionists look at the way your body *reacts* to the carbs,

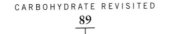

rather than at the number of sugar molecules. The principal tool for measuring this is the glycemic index (GI), which indicates how quickly a food turns into glucose, a blood sugar that's your body's preferred fuel. Foods that are quickly digested and turned to glucose are referred to as being *high-glycemic*, while those that are more slowly transformed are called *low-glycemic*.

When you eat high-glycemic foods, the quick rush of glucose that results prompts your body to use straight glucose for energy, rather than a mixture of glucose and fat. So none of your fat reserves are burned off as fuel. Furthermore, since any fat you've just eaten along with the carbs is not needed as an immediate energy source, it's added to your flabby, blubbery reserves.

From there it gets worse: Since your body digests high-glycemic foods quickly, they empty out of your stomach faster. And as we said earlier, this releases a rush of glucose into your bloodstream, which in turn signals the release of a surge of the hormone insulin that directs your body to use the glucose for its immediate energy needs and to store any excess in muscle cells. This subsequently creates a sharp dip in your blood sugar. So your body then signals its need for more fuel by kicking off a hunger response. Your hunger returns faster and more intensely following a high-glycemic meal.

It's sort of a vicious cycle. Shampoo, rinse, repeat, until you've either gotten too fat to see your ding-dong or developed insulin resistance (a precursor of diabetes type 2 and heart disease). Or, if you're really lucky, both.

INDEX FUN

The glycemic index assigns all carbohydrate-containing foods a number representing how quickly your body turns them to glucose. In general, the lower the number, the better. Foods with GIs of 55 or lower cause only a small change in blood sugar, but those with GIs of 70 or above shoot your glucose level into outer space.

Here's a list of foods and how they rank.

GI RATINGS OF COMMON FOODS

FRUITS
Cherries	32
Plum	34
Grapefruit	36
Pear	51
Apple	52
Apple juice	58
Grapes	62
Orange	62
Grapefruit juice	69
Orange juice	74
Banana	76
Fruit cocktail	79
Raisins	91
Pineapple	94
Watermelon	103

DAIRY PRODUCTS
Yogurt (artificially sweetened)	20
Whole milk	39
Skim milk	46
Low-fat ice cream	71
Ice cream	87

LEGUMES
Lentils	41
Kidney beans	42
Split peas	45
Lima beans	46
Chickpeas	47
Pinto beans	55
Baked beans	69

VEGETABLES
Peas	68
Sweet potato	77
Corn	78
Carrots	101
Potato	121

GRAINS AND PASTAS
Barley	36
Rye	48
Spaghetti	59
Wheat	59
Linguine	65
Brown rice	79
White rice	81
Instant rice	128

SOUPS
Tomato	54
Lentil	63
Split Pea	86

CEREALS
All-Bran	60
Oat bran	78
Shredded wheat	99
Puffed wheat	105
Cheerios	106
Rice Krispies	117
Corn flakes	119

SNACKS
Peanuts	21
Chocolate	70
Potato chips	77
Oatmeal cookies	79
Popcorn	79
Corn chips	105
Vanilla wafers	110

Jelly beans	114	Angel food cake	95
Rice cakes	117	Croissant	96
		Doughnut	108
SUGARS		Waffle	109
Fructose	32		
Lactose	65	**BREADS**	
Sucrose	92	Hamburger bun	87
Honey	104	White bread	99
Glucose	138	Whole wheat bread	99
Maltose	150	Bagel	103
		Kaiser roll	104
PASTRIES			
Sponge cake	66		
Bran muffin	85		

As you can see, some simple carbohydrates like fruits and dairy products rate low on the index (which is good), while complex carbs like breads can rank pretty high (which is bad, except in one instance, which we'll explain in the next section).

Though sugar content is generally a good indicator of a food's ranking, other factors can affect its GI rating. For instance, while a food may be high in sugar, the other nutrients it contains may slow down your body's digestion of it. Protein, fat, and fiber content slow down the rate of digestion of any given food, which means it takes longer for glucose to hit your bloodstream. Another factor is the size of the individual particles of the food. For instance, instant oatmeal has a higher glycemic index number than slow-cooking oatmeal, and refined flour also is turned to glucose faster than whole grain flour, because the processing that the former foods undergo breaks them down into smaller particles and decreases their fiber content.

A RISING TIDE LIFTS ALL MUSCLES

There is only one point in your day when we recommend high-glycemic-index carbohydrate, and that's following exercise. A good workout leaves your muscles drained of their stored glycogen, their preferred source of energy. A lack of glycogen causes your body to use two other sources of energy: fat and amino acids. No problem with the fat, but where do you think you get those amino acids? That's right—from the protein in your muscles.

Make no mistake, this is a state of emergency for your body. Fortunately, it's easily remedied. The faster you throw carbohydrate into your stomach, the faster your body produces insulin. Insulin does two amazing things immediately after exercise: It stops protein breakdown and starts protein synthesis. Some studies have shown that adding protein to the postexercise meal increases this tide of insulin, and some haven't. All we can say for sure is that carbohydrate is the most important part of the postexercise meal.

And the higher the glycemic index rating of the carbohydrate, the faster this process begins. That's why many post-workout meal-replacement supplements include maltodextrin, an easily digested carb made from cornstarch. As you saw in the list of glycemic index rankings, maltose, found in maltodextrin, has an even higher GI number than glucose does.

In chapter 10, we'll take a closer look at pre- and postexercise nutrition.

Putting
Together
the Food Plan

*T*he T diet involves three important calculations: metabolism, or the number of calories you burn on a daily basis; goals, or whether you want to lose fat, gain muscle, or maintain your current weight while changing your body composition; and your daily protein requirements.

METABOLISM

Before we can tell you how to personalize the T diet, you need to figure out how many calories it takes for you to keep the body you have right now. Use this formula.

LINE 1: Your weight in pounds = 165

LINE 2: Your basic calorie needs
Line 1 _____ × 11 (the number
of calories you'd use just lying
on the couch all day, without
getting up or eating anything) = 1,815

We presume you're doing more with your life than fasting motionless on the sofa. That's why you have to consider the effect that your activity level has on your metabolic factor. We've created three categories with which to rate your current activity level.

1. Consider yourself **MOSTLY SEDENTARY** if you have a desk job, don't exercise regularly, and don't have any hobbies or other activities that keep you on your feet for any appreciable amount of time each day.

2. **MODERATELY ACTIVE** describes you if you have a job that involves activity beyond sitting at a computer or behind the wheel of a car or truck. This category also includes the guy who takes a long walk or bike ride each day, or spends his weekends doing yard work or building additions to his house. Still not sure if you belong in this category? Use this yardstick: If you spend at least 2 hours a day on your feet, whether for work or play, or if you have a daily hour-long exercise routine, you can consider yourself moderately active.

3. **DEDICATED EXERCISER OR ATHLETE** describes you if you do some sort of high-intensity exercise almost every day, or if you've lifted weights 3 or 4 days a week for at least a year. The weight lifter's metabolism burns calories at a relatively high rate even at rest because of his muscle mass, while the guy who plays basketball or hockey regularly burns up a lot of calories simply from the activity itself.

Age also makes a difference in your metabolic factor. Everyone starts to slow down postadolescence—this is biologically programmed and occurs across all species as a normal part of the aging process. By the time you hit 30, inactivity starts to take a toll on your metabolic rate, to the tune of about 1 percent a year. It's possible to reverse this at any age with muscle-building exercise, and our T workouts certainly will have that effect. But we need to give you some figures to start with, so here goes.

	UNDER 30 YEARS OLD	30–40 YEARS OLD	OVER 40 YEARS OLD
Mostly sedentary	30%	25%	20%
Moderately active	40%	35%	30%
Dedicated exerciser or athlete	50%	45%	40%

Multiply the appropriate percentage by your basic calorie needs to calculate your metabolic factor.

> **LINE 3:** Your metabolic factor
> Line 2 1815 × 40 %   = 726

You can now determine the number of calories you need in your diet just to maintain the status quo. Add your basic calorie needs to your metabolic factor.

> **LINE 4:** Your maintenance diet
> Line 2 1815 + Line 3 726   = 2541

GOALS

Some guys who pick up this book are happy with the number on the scale and just want to change their body composition—build more muscle and shed some fat. Others want to gain or lose. Since 2 pounds of fat equals 7,000 calories, you'll need to subtract 1,000 calories a day from your diet to lose that much each week (that is, 1,000 calories × 7 days = 7,000 calories subtracted, hence 2 pounds lost). Add 500 calories a day, and the T diet and workout should combine to put about a pound of muscle a week on your frame.

So let's say you're a 45-year-old, 230-pound guy who wants to get leaner. You're sedentary now, so you give yourself a metabolic factor of 20 percent, which brings you to a maintenance diet of about 3,000 calories a day. Subtract 1,000 calories, and you see you can eat about 2,000 calories a day and lose 2 pounds a week.

Or let's say you're a very active 150-pound 25-year-old who wants to gain muscular weight. You add 500 calories to a 2,475-calorie-a-day maintenance diet, and you get 2,975, or 3,000 if you round it upward. Eat that many calories every day, and you should add a pound of muscle a week.

Finally, maybe you're a 35-year-old, 180-pound guy who's fairly active and doesn't want to gain or lose weight—just maybe shave an inch off your waistline and add some beef to your chest and shoulders. Run the numbers, and you see that your maintenance calorie intake is about 2,700 daily calories.

We must add one stipulation to your calorie calculations: Keep your calorie intake at 2,000 or above even if the math indicates that you need fewer. Dipping below 2,000 calories per day can compromise both your testosterone levels and your ability to build muscle. Don't worry, you'll still lose lard—you'll just do it without starving yourself or your muscles.

PROTEIN

Remember, we told you that the T plan calls for 2 grams of protein per kilogram of body weight. This comes out to 0.91 gram per pound. So multiply your present weight by 0.91, and that's your daily protein requirement. If you weigh 230 pounds, this gives you about 209 grams of protein a day. (You'll adjust this figure up or down at the end of the program, based on how much muscle you've gained and how much body fat you've lost. We'll explain all that in chapter 17.)

NUMBERS GAME

Now that you have your daily calorie total and your protein total, the rest of your T diet falls into place.

Let's go back to our 230-pound 45-year-old who wants to slim down. We already calculated that he should eat about 2,000 calories per day in order to lose 2 pounds of fat a week, and that he needs 209 grams of protein. Now we need to figure out what proportions of his diet will be protein, fat, and carbohydrate.

A Few Words about Weight Gain

In the old days, a guy who wanted to gain weight would go to his local "health" food store and buy a big can of weight-gainer powder, which would add about 1,000 calories a day to his diet, most of it sugar. And he'd gain weight all right, but damn near all of it would be fat.

We know better now. If you want to get bigger without getting fatter, you're much better off adding 500 calories a day to your diet. Combined with a good weight-training program, that should add about a pound of muscle a week to your frame.

In truth, we hesitate to promise that you'll bulk even that much—9 pounds of muscle in 9 weeks is a lot. We couldn't find anyone for our pilot study who was interested in gaining weight (that's what happens when you start a program in January), so we don't know that these theoretical results are achievable. We think about what 9 pounds of muscle would look like on a 150-pound guy—an inch on his chest and thighs, maybe a half-inch on his arms and calves—and believe that it's possible in 9 weeks. Is it realistic? We honestly aren't sure.

In theory, it's also possible to gain muscle even faster—up to 2 pounds per week for short periods—but people who pull this off tend to be clustered suspiciously in Body for Life competitions.

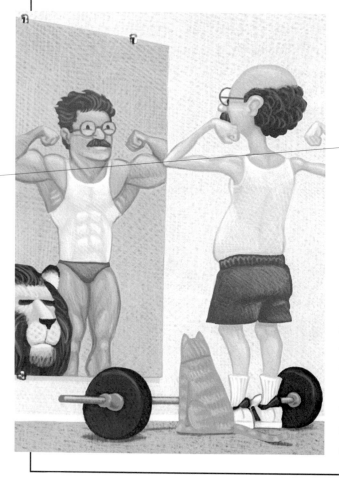

A gram of protein, on average, has 4 calories, so we see he'll get 836 calories a day from protein. That's about 42 percent of his total calories (836 divided by 2,000 equals 42 percent, which we'll round down to 40 for simplicity).

That leaves 60 percent of his calories to split evenly between fat and carbohydrates, which means he'll get 30 percent of his daily calories from each. So now we know he'll get 600 calories (2,000 times 0.3) from fat and 600 from carbohydrate. A gram of fat has 9 calories, so he'll get 67 grams daily. A gram of carbohydrate has an average of 4 calories, so the remaining 600 calories of his diet will comprise 150 grams of carbs.

Now let's look at our 150-pounder who wants to gain muscular weight. He starts with 137 grams of protein, which is 548 calories, or about 18 percent of his 3,000-calorie daily intake. So now he should eat 41 percent fat and 41 percent carbohydrate.

The 180-pound guy will eat 164 grams of protein. That's 656 calories, or about 25 percent of his daily 2,700 calories. The other three-quarters of his diet is split evenly between fat and carbohydrate.

To make all this simpler, let's put it into a chart.

	GUY #1	GUY #2	GUY #3
Age	45	25	35
Weight	230	150	180
Metabolic factor	20%	50%	35%
Goal	2 lb/wk fat loss (−1,000 calories)	1 lb/wk muscle (+500 calories)	Weight maintenance
Daily calories	2,000 calories	3,000 calories	2,700 calories
Daily protein grams	209 g	137 g	164 g
Daily protein calories (g × 4)	836 calories	548 calories	656 calories
Daily protein % (rounded off)	40%	18%	25%
Daily fat/carb %	30%/30%	41%/41%	38%/38%

	GUY #1	GUY #2	GUY #3
Daily fat/carb calories	600/600 calories	1,230/1,230 calories	1,026/1,026 calories
Daily fat grams (fat calories ÷ 9)	67 g	137 g	114 g
Daily carb grams (carb calories ÷ 4)	150 g	308 g	257 g

THE GREAT WEIGHT DEBATE

Considering that the majority of Americans—60 percent—are overweight, we suspect that most guys who buy this book will relate to our hypothetical Mr. 230, who wants to lose his gut or his beer belly or his spare tire or his love handles or whatever else he jokingly calls his midsection in lieu of the medical term, *disgusting fat*. So we're going to play to our audience, and spend some more time talking about diet and fat loss. In the past few years, we've seen specialists in fitness and nutrition divide themselves into two philosophical camps when this subject arises. These opposing camps are *energy balance* versus *macronutrient balance*.

ENERGY BALANCE. This group believes that your body composition is determined solely by the amount of energy you take in (the number of calories in your food) and the amount you expend (the number of calories you burn through digestion, daily activities, and exercise). Most of the published research supports this philosophy, so we have to confess that we're mostly in this camp, although we emphasize that some phenomena can't be explained by energy balance alone.

The energy-balance argument goes like this: No matter how you trick up a diet, the bottom line is that, with some highly technical exceptions still being investigated, a calorie is a calorie. So whether you lose your gut on the Paleolithic diet or on the Atkins diet or by eating only llamas, the diet works not because you've cut all the carbohydrate but simply because you have limited your dietary choices and are therefore eating less overall.

Generally, the foods that people tend to overeat compulsively are high-glycemic carbohydrates combined with fat and salt. A French study published in the *International Journal of Eating Disorders* in 2001 found that a craving for sweets is a sign that you're tired, while a craving for salty foods or milk products usually means that you're hungry. Also, the study found, men tend to have stronger food cravings when they're happy. It's no surprise, then, that when guys are hungry, happy, and hanging out—Super Bowl Sunday comes to mind—we keep eating past the point at which we would ordinarily stop. And the foods we eat—pizza following an appetizer of potato chips with sour cream dip, all washed down with beer—are the worst ones for our waistlines.

If we had to guess, we'd say 99 percent of nutritionists and researchers believe in the calories-in/calories-out theory of weight control. But that still leaves 1 percent who think other factors play a bigger role. So what could account for increases or reductions in body fat, if not calories?

MACRONUTRIENT BALANCE. That 1 percent of scientists thinks the answer is the drastic reduction of particular macronutrients—in other words, diets that are extremely low carb or incredibly low fat. For instance, in chapter 6 of *Dr. Atkins' New Diet Revolution*, the author cites a long list of studies, dating back 50 years, showing that extremely low carbohydrate diets induce weight loss and fat loss that can't be explained by the calories-in/calories-out energy-balance theory.

The energy-balance camp is quick to point out that diets in which people cut out or severely restrict entire macronutrients tend to fail in the long run. The Atkins diet may actually prove them right. We know the book has sold millions of copies, so in theory there are millions of people out there who have tried that super-low-carb diet. If it's successful, there should be millions of people who have lost weight on the diet and kept it off. That doesn't appear to be the case.

The National Weight Control Registry surveyed its members, all of whom had lost at least 30 pounds and kept them off for at least a year, to see how many of them had used an Atkins-like diet to achieve their weight loss. It discovered that just 7.6 percent of the 2,681 members had followed that type of low-carbohydrate plan. So even though we do have before us a sampling of people who did lose weight with a super-low-carb diet, the small overall number—just 200 or so people out of almost 2,700 successful dieters—suggests that such a diet is by no means the most effective slim-down strategy. And let's not forget that this tells us nothing about how many people *tried* a low-carb diet and didn't succeed with it. Nor, for that matter, does it tell us what even the successful dieters looked like afterward. For all we know, they could've ended up with nice, slim bodies almost completely devoid of muscle tissue. That's not what we're after on the T plan.

In *The Protein Power Lifeplan*, Drs. Michael and Mary Dan Eades recall the case of a patient who wondered why she'd lost only 4 pounds on a virtually carb-free diet. When they looked at her daily food intake—including breakfasts of four eggs and five or six pieces of bacon and sausage—they saw she was eating more than 5,000 calories a day. That's an awful lot of calories in. How the hell had she even lost 4 pounds?

That's not to let Ornish and Pritikin and the super low fat fanatics off the hook. We've seen some studies that looked at whether anyone can comply with a diet like this. One such study, published in *Archives of Family Medicine*, put 10 volunteers on an Ornish-type vegetarian diet, with fewer than 10 percent of calories coming from fat. A year later, fat loss ranged from ¼ pound (that's not a typo) to 26 pounds. And the subjects' cholesterol levels were unchanged. Furthermore, just 1 of the 10 subjects had managed to follow the diet to the letter. If you're trying to make a case for very low fat diets, one is a pretty damn lonely number.

So high-carb diets aren't the answer. And the ultra low fat plans don't work either, in part because they're too hard to follow. That's why we started with the Mediterranean diet, with its healthful use of monounsaturated fats, and then modified it with animal protein and low-glycemic carbs to produce the best muscle-building effect when combined with our T workouts. We know the T diet and T workout are effective in combination. The guys in our pilot study who were trying to lose tonnage dropped it steadily and in line with our expectations, based on the calories in the diet.

Why Not Diet Pills?

For starters, how 'bout the fact that they can kill you?

The ones that actually work usually do so by kicking the metabolic process into superhigh gear, with unpredictable results. You may recall that the supposed weight-loss godsend fen-phen (a cocktail of dexfenfluramine and fenfluramine, sold under the brand name Redux) was pulled from pharmacy shelves in 1997 after studies tied the drug to permanent heart-valve damage in an unacceptable number of patients.

Even highly publicized Meridia (sibutramine) can have negative side effects, including severe, potentially dangerous blood-pressure spikes. All those disclaimers on TV ads and product packages are there for a reason, after all, and they should be enough to make any prospective Meridia user think twice.

Even when they're not damaging your heart or shooting your blood pressure through the roof, drugs just don't seem as effective as diet-and-behavior modification. We're going to quote a study involving women here—don't get nasty about it, because (a) gender isn't the point in this case and (b) this just proves our basic contention that when the medical establishment wants to study weight loss, it usually studies women. Anyway, the women in one segment of a 1-year trial were assigned to groups that received either Meridia or Meridia plus information on healthy eating. The women on Meridia alone lost an average of 4.1 percent of their initial weights. Not bad. But the women in the Meridia-plus-lifestyle-modification group lost an average of 10.8 percent.

So unless you are morbidly obese and need immediate intervention, don't grab a drug. Go grab a dumbbell instead.

Some of the guys, though, surprised us by losing more or less than we'd expected. And that brings up another point: It's impossible to know in advance exactly what effect a diet and workout program will have on you. The metabolic calculations we use are just an educated guess. A guy who starts to drop a few may find that he becomes a lot more active in his day-to-day life, so he gets a multiplier effect. In fact, a University of Alabama-Birmingham study published in the *Journal of Applied Physiology* in 2000 found that older adults increased daily activity by an average of 23 minutes during a 26-week weight-training program. That's 23 minutes over and above the amount of time they spent actually lifting weights. The subjects got all the results you'd expect in a weight-training study: increased strength (36 percent), increased muscle mass (4.4 pounds), decreased fat (6.8 pounds), and increased resting metabolism (6.8 percent). The surprise was the extra time they spent up and moving.

But that's a nice surprise, isn't it?

CHAPTER

IO

When You Eat,
and Why It Matters

*T*he idea of "three squares a day" is great . . . if you're in prison. There, your days are a blur of weight lifting, showers, staring at walls, more weight lifting, more showers, negotiating with that guy who's had his eye on you since the first shower. . . . It's a wonder you find the time to eat at all!

It's funny, though. In a sense, we *have* been in prison, many of us— imprisoned by traditional notions of when and what we should eat: breakfast at 7:00 A.M., lunch at noon, dinner at 6:00 P.M.. The fact is, a regular guy who hopes to get the most out of himself can't settle for three meals a day. He needs five.

Why? We like to borrow the following analogy from Dan Benardot, Ph.D., a nutrition researcher at Georgia State University who has worked with U.S. Olympic teams.

Suppose you're driving from New York to Florida and you want to get there as efficiently as possible. You could do it one of three ways.

1. You could fill up your car in New York, drive until you get to the last drop of gas, hope that you have enough fumes left to get to a

gas station, fill up on whatever's available when you happen to run out, then drive until your tank is empty again.

2. Before you start out, you could get all the gas you need for the entire trip. This would involve rigging your car with extra gas tanks and filling them up the night before you leave.

3. You could stop at regular intervals on the way (usually when your tank is about three-quarters empty), fill up with the best-quality gas available, and continue on.

To all but the biggest risk-takers, option 3 seems like the best idea. Not only do you always have plenty of fuel in reserve but you never end up at the mercy of price gougers selling a low-grade product. (Like, what if you're driving a car that requires premium, but you get to the service station and they only have the 87 octane?) Option 1 is almost sure to make you a worst-possible-scenario poster child: Your car finally crawls to a dead stop in the middle of an overpass crossing a mosquito-infested alligator swamp. As for option 2? It's way too dangerous to drive around with all that extra fuel. For one thing, the added weight would make the car unwieldy and more expensive to drive. For another, one fender-bender and . . . well, you certainly would make the evening news in whatever town you were in when you stopped existing.

Now imagine that the car is your body, and the drive from New York to Florida is just a normal, stress-filled day in your life. The gas, obviously, is your food.

Option 1 is the way most guys eat. We push ourselves until we're starving, then we grab whatever we can find and call it a meal. It could come from a candy machine, a drive-thru window, or that ball of aluminum foil in the back of the fridge, the contents of which we can't identify but assume to be mostly protein in origin. There's absolutely no quality control here. When we're out of gas, we don't have the option of selecting the best grade of fuel. Whatever will make the engines run is what we put in our tanks.

Option 2 is even worse. Unfortunately, in our experience, it's the option of choice for many heavy guys: They're on what amounts to the

One-Meal-a-Day Diet. They skip breakfast, grab lunch on the fly, snack on anything they happen to find lying around, then gorge themselves at dinner, eating the caloric equivalent of three or four meals in one sitting. Indigestion sets in, so they sleep fitfully, have trouble waking up in the morning, skip breakfast again, and start the process anew.

As time goes on, these guys build ever-larger "spare tanks" of reserve fuel in the form of fat. And, just as it would be dangerous to drive cross-country with a few hundred gallons of gas sloshing around in the trunk of your car, so it is risky to walk around all day holding all this fat in your abdomen (the most likely storage site). Heart disease is one expected result, but adult-onset diabetes and any number of cancers could come along for the ride. And it almost goes without saying that the extra weight makes life difficult; it's tough to maneuver, impossible to squeeze into tight spaces, and a terrible burden on the parts of your body that have to carry the load: your lower back, hips, knees, ankles, feet. Finally, if you're called upon to perform at an unexpected level of physical output—say, shoveling snow—you're really asking for trouble.

This brings us back to option 3. The most efficient way to fuel a car or a human is to make regular stops for the highest-quality fuel. That means breakfast, mid-morning snack, lunch, mid-afternoon snack, and dinner.

All the meals are important, of course, but two matter more than the others.

BREAKFAST: THE KING OF ALL MEALS

Over the years, we've seen intriguing studies showing an inverse link between breakfast and obesity. People were more likely to be obese if they skipped breakfast. Looking deeper, cereal usually had a lot to do with it: The more cereal the subjects in these studies ate, the less likely they were to be obese.

But breakfast seems to play an even bigger role in total health. California Department of Public Health officials following a group of subjects in Alameda County since 1965 have found seven lifestyle habits that translate to health and longevity. The first six seem obvious: exercise, weight control, moderate drinking, a full night's sleep, a cigarette-free lifestyle, and eating planned meals (not just randomly snacking, in other words).

The seventh, however, is the surprise: The healthiest, longest-living people eat breakfast.

Breakfast on the T diet will be similar to all the other meals; the goal is to start your day with a ratio of protein, fat, and carbohydrate that stays close to the one you're trying to follow throughout the diet.

It's by far the most important meal on the plan. A hearty breakfast helps prevent food cravings later in the day. It gives your body protein to work with, preventing it from cannibalizing your biceps to get the amino acids it needs to keep your systems running. And it stabilizes your blood sugar, giving you a source of steady energy to start your day.

Plus, as a bonus, it helps you outlive people who don't eat breakfast. How cool is that?

POST-WORKOUT PROVISIONS:
THE WINDOW OF OPPORTUNITY

For as long as any of us have been working out, we've heard that the best way to build muscle is to take in as much protein as possible as soon as possible after our workouts. Science has traditionally scoffed at this idea, chalking it up to bodybuilding mythology. After all, the body doesn't use protein for energy during a workout, so why would it need protein to recover after a workout? The key to postexercise recovery, scientists contended, was carbohydrate, which they sold us as a two-for-the-price-of-one postexercise problem solver: It supposedly provided the nutrient your body needed to replenish its stores of glycogen (its "preferred" energy source, stored carbohydrate), and it stimulated insulin, the hormone that speeds nutrients to muscles for refuel and repair.

Muscleheads laughed at the idea that carbohydrate could be more important than protein following a workout. After all, they reasoned, these scientists had been strutting around for decades with a carb-on for protein, saying no one needs extra amino acids for muscle growth. And these were the same pencil necks who insisted that steroids didn't build muscle and who stuck by that claim till the mid-1990s, almost 4 decades after Eastern European athletes turned the sports world upside down by using anabolic drugs. How could you trust anything that came from a bunch of cardio cultists who habitually oversold the benefits of aerobic exercise and dismissed the wonders of weight lifting?

The musclehead community reasoned that if the idea is to increase protein synthesis—the conversion of food to muscle—why in the world wouldn't you give your body protein to convert?

Of course, building new muscle through protein synthesis is only half of the postexercise story. The other half is preventing protein degradation—that is, the tearing down of the muscle you already have.

Insulin prevents protein breakdown, and after exercise your body will release more insulin with a combination of carbohydrate and protein than it will with carbohydrate alone. So if you want to build the most muscle with the least muscle breakdown, you need a combination of carbohydrate and protein as soon as possible following exercise.

Any of the meals in the T plan should serve you well after a workout. Just make sure you eat them ASAP.

We can't say this strongly enough: Don't dawdle.
Go straight from the weight room to the dining room.

Lost time is lost muscle.

GONNA TAKE A SUPPLEMENTAL JOURNEY?

Having just learned how crucial it is to get protein and carbs immediately after a workout, you might ask yourself, "Wouldn't it be easier—not to mention faster—to just grab a protein shake or bar, as long as it also has plenty of carbs?"

The answer is, supplements are the devil's work. They're developed by profoundly evil men with cloven hooves beneath their white lab coats, marketed by corporate myrmidons, and consumed by deluded narcissists who've sold their souls to GNC. Every evil of modern life can be attributed to the supplement industry.

Sorry. For a minute there, we accidentally channeled the thoughts of the last nutritionist we spoke to.

To tell you the truth, we don't have a problem with meal-replacement supplements. They're convenient, and they may make you feel that you're serious about improving your health and physique. They're another level of commitment, along with regular workouts and adhering to a healthy diet. Plus, getting your post-workout carbs and protein in the liquid form of a shake means you get nutrients to your muscles faster, and you know we're in favor of that.

But the fact that nutrients reach your muscles faster doesn't necessarily mean that your muscles will grow faster. We don't know whether a shake or bar is any more or less effective than a turkey sandwich at promoting protein synthesis and preventing protein degradation. Most studies on meal supplements are funded by the supplement companies themselves, and to our knowledge, no manufacturers have tested their products against whole food. They've only compared supplements with other supplements—a liquid-protein-and-carbohydrate combination versus liquid carbohydrate alone, for example.

Our guess—and taking a guess is all we can really do at this moment in nutritional history—is that the main benefit of protein supplements over food is that convenience factor, especially immediately after a workout. We feel safe in concluding that they aren't dangerous in any known way, so if you file them under "Can't hurt, might help," you're unlikely to be disappointed—whether you use them or not.

If you do decide to use them, we recommend that you limit the meal replacements in your diet to one per day. Science is just beginning to unravel the mysteries of food, and until we see a study showing that fake food is better than the real stuff, we like to err on the side of the latter. So even though supplement manufacturers like to toss a hobo's stew of vitamins and other nutrients into their products, we still want you to get most of your calories from actual food.

Make sure you take that nutrient stew into account when you plan your other meals. Shakes and bars bundle a lot of calories into a very small package, so they can be very helpful if you have trouble eating enough food to meet your caloric needs. But if, like most guys, you're

"MY WIFE IS JEALOUS"

Like many participants, Mike Smith was "shocked" at how much flab he lost—even though he "fudged a little."

On his motivation for going on the T plan: *"We had a baby in April, and I'd put on about 10 pounds of weight too. I wanted to get the weight off. Much to my shock, I lost 33 pounds. I dropped below 230 pounds for the first time since my sophomore year of college."*

On others' reactions: *"My daughter said, 'Daddy, you don't have a belly anymore.' My wife is jealous. . . . At budget meetings at work, everybody's remarking, 'Something's different about you.'"*

On the T plan's ease of use: *"You got to eat foods you like, throughout the day. . . . The food doesn't take long to prepare, either."*

On the physical benefits: *"Around the wallyball court [indoor volleyball played on a racquetball court], my game has improved. It's high intensity, with a lot of diving and jumping and spiking. I'm able to get to shots that would've been difficult in the past. I seem to have better agility and hand-eye coordination."*

Bottom line: *"The program has changed my life in that it got me to realize the symptoms of unhealthy eating. When you have a couple of Big Macs once or twice a week, it affects your body. I just don't do it anymore. I recognize that there's good food I can eat and still feel satisfied."*

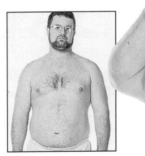

MIKE SMITH, 35, 6' 2"

VITAL STATS		BEFORE T PLAN	AFTER T PLAN
	WEIGHT	262 lb	234 lb
	WAIST	43½"	39"
	BENCH PRESS	255 lb	270 lb

more likely to consume too many calories than to eat too few, you have to remember to include any supplements when you calculate your daily diet.

For instance, if you have a post-workout shake that contains 40 grams of protein (160 calories) and 80 grams of carbs (320 calories), that's 480 calories. On a 2,000-calorie-a-day diet, that one shake is close to 25 percent of your daily total. And it doesn't include any fat, so you have to either include some fat in the shake or make up for it at other meals. We simplified this a bit for you in chapter 11, creating three different meal-replacement shakes with different ratios of protein, carbs, and fat so you can see how this would work. And a ready-to-drink shake or a bar may actually be easier to account for than a post-workout snack of, say, a banana, because the nutrient content is printed right on the package. (Chiquita hasn't yet figured out how to fit Nutrition Facts on that tiny sticker.)

Unfortunately, the calories in a protein bar are so densely packed that you may still feel hungry after eating it. After all, it takes only a few seconds to wolf it down. Another potential drawback is that protein bars have been known to cause gastrointestinal distress in some people. No one is sure why, but some researchers speculate that it's due to a common ingredient called glycerol, a sugar alcohol that's often used in place of carbs. Others think it's because some bars contain lactose, the main sugar in milk. Some think it's the high protein content that can lead to trouble down below. At any rate, if you find that a particular type of bar gives you digestive problems, switch brands. Experimentation is the only way to know for sure which product will work for you.

STAY HUNGRY, BUT DON'T TRAIN HUNGRY

We told you that breakfast and your postexercise fare are the most crucial meals of the day. The rankings among your other three feedings are mostly equal, although your pre-exercise meal may deserve a bit more consideration.

That's because you won't get as good a workout if you're ravenously

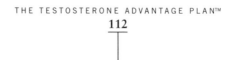

hungry or so stuffed that you're sluggish. You want enough food in your stomach to prevent hunger pangs, but not so much that an undigested mass of it prevents you from pushing yourself in the weight room.

We think this is fairly simple to arrange.

A good rule of thumb is to exercise 1 hour after a snack or 2 hours after a meal.

So if you like to exercise in the morning, we recommend a snack as soon as you wake up, followed an hour later by a workout, followed immediately by a full meal—in this case, breakfast. Or if you like to work out before lunch, just make sure you have your mid-morning snack 1 hour before you hit the weight room. And if you're an after-work exerciser, time it so you train 1 hour after your mid-afternoon snack.

The
1-Week
Meal Planner

*T*hese plans are models for anyone using the T diet. If you want to get trimmer, see the plan for the 230-pounder ("heavyweight"), and adjust the calories and protein in each meal to meet your targets.

The meal plan for the 180-pounder ("cruiserweight") shows how an average guy who's in decent shape can use the T diet to change his body composition without gaining or losing significant amounts of weight.

Finally, the guy who wants to put on a few pounds can use the diet for the 150-pounder ("welterweight") as a model of how to get enough calories in a day to accomplish that goal.

Adhere as closely as possible to the appropriate grocery list and daily menus, brand names included. Check calorie and macronutrient contents before making substitutions. Pay attention to product labels. To wash it all down, drink 12 ounces of water with each meal, plus the specified beverages.

The initial 2 weeks will be the hardest simply because it will probably be a drastic change from the way you've been eating. Once you adjust, you'll find that you're eating a lot and you're never hungry.

Enough of the windup. Here's the pitch.

Shake It Up

Here are three protein shakes designed for guys to use in this program. Most of us drink them after workouts and as occasional meal replacements on days when we don't exercise. They make it easy to ensure that we get enough protein each day. But we want to stress that convenience and necessity are separate issues. Until someone performs a well-controlled study showing that protein supplements produce better muscle gains than real food does, we'll remain on the fence about whether a guy actually needs them to achieve the best possible results from his workouts.

Any name-brand whey protein should work fine as the basis of these shakes. Two that have good reputations are EAS and Twinlab. The whey protein is usually packaged with a plastic scoop for measuring. Check the label to see how many grams are in one scoop; in most cases, there are 25 grams.

230-POUND GUY (HEAVYWEIGHT)

½ cup frozen vanilla yogurt

½ cup 1% milk

1 tablespoon + 1 teaspoon peanut butter

1 tablespoon unsweetened cocoa powder

45 grams whey protein

YIELDS ABOUT 10 OUNCES; CALORIES: 480; PROTEIN: 47 G; FAT: 16 G; CARBOHYDRATE: 37 G

180-POUND GUY (CRUISERWEIGHT)

2 cups 1% milk

¾ cup frozen strawberries

1 tablespoon + 1 teaspoon olive oil

½ cup strawberry yogurt

19 grams (about ¾ scoop) whey protein

YIELDS ABOUT 27 OUNCES; CALORIES: 609; PROTEIN: 39 G; FAT: 25 G; CARBOHYDRATE: 57 G

150-POUND GUY (WELTERWEIGHT)

⅓ cup heavy cream

1 cup frozen strawberries

1 cup strawberry yogurt

38 grams (about 1½ scoops) whey protein

YIELDS ABOUT 20 OUNCES; CALORIES: 690; PROTEIN: 38 G; FAT: 30 G; CARBOHYDRATE: 67 G

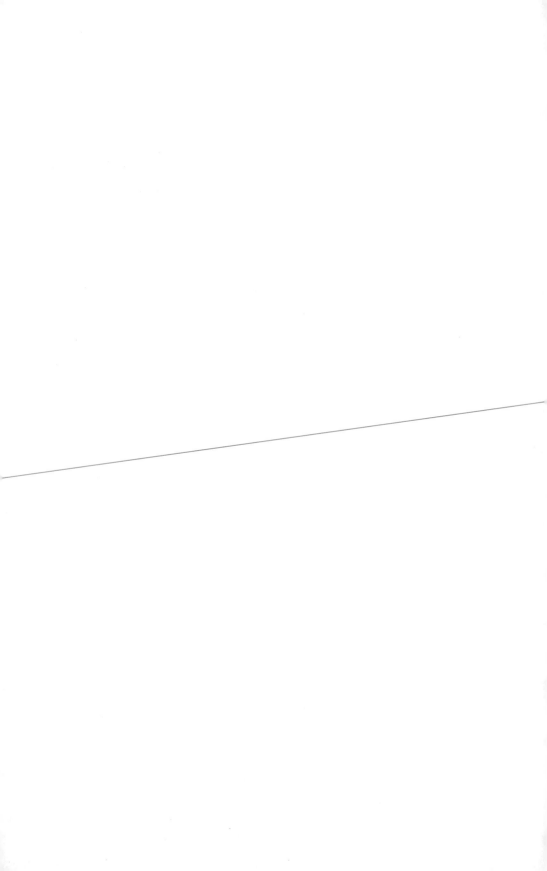

HEAVYWEIGHT

GROCERY LIST

ONE-TIME ITEMS

Olive oil

Canola oil

Dry-roasted peanuts

Soy sauce

Minced garlic

Ketchup

Mustard

Dill pickles

Sweet pickle relish

Brown sugar

Fresh ginger

Italian seasoning

Salt

Ground black pepper

Lemon juice

Fat-free Miracle Whip
salad dressing

Lite syrup

WEEKLY ITEMS

1½ gallons of 1% milk

1 pint of 2% chocolate
milk

1 package of string
cheese

5 24-ounce containers
of 1% cottage cheese

1 16-ounce bag
of shredded low-fat
Cheddar cheese

1 package of Cheddar
cheese slices

1 small block
of Parmesan cheese

2 ounces of feta cheese

4 ounces of goat cheese

2 8-ounce containers
of Egg Beaters
or egg substitute

1 container of full-fat
fruit yogurt

5 6-ounce cans
of water-packed tuna

2 loaves of thin
multigrain bread

8 multigrain rolls

½ pound of spinach

5 tomatoes

1 white onion

1 pound of asparagus

1 cantaloupe

1 pineapple or 2 cups
of pineapple chunks

2 peaches

1 1-pound bag of frozen
stir-fry vegetables

1 pound of green beans

1 1-pound bag of frozen
mixed vegetables

1 box of frozen
multigrain waffles

1 pound of turkey
Italian sausage

2 packages of turkey
sausage links

1½ pounds of boneless,
skinless chicken
breasts

1½ pounds of fat-free
turkey lunchmeat

4 6- to 7-ounce salmon
fillets

1 pound of raw shrimp

2 pounds of T-bone
steak

3 pounds of at least
90%-lean ground beef

1 container of pesto

1 box of dried penne

1 box of rolled oats

1 box of Shredded
Wheat and Bran

1 package of chili
seasoning

1 15-ounce can
of kidney beans

1 8-ounce can
of tomato juice

1 28-ounce and
1 16-ounce can
of diced tomatoes

1 box of saltines

BREAKFAST

1 cup of Shredded Wheat and Bran with ¾ cup of 1% milk

5 links of turkey breakfast sausage

CALORIES: 590; PROTEIN: 43 G; FAT: 26 G; CARBS: 46 G

SNACK 1

1 ounce of dry-roasted peanuts

1 cup of 1% milk

1 cup of 1% cottage cheese

CALORIES: 439; PROTEIN: 43 G; FAT: 19 G; CARBS: 24 G

LUNCH

Sandwich made with 2 slices of multigrain bread, 1 tablespoon of fat-free Miracle Whip, 6 ounces of fat-free turkey lunchmeat, ½ cup of spinach, and 2 slices of tomato

CALORIES: 279; PROTEIN: 30 G; FAT: 3 G; CARBS: 33 G

SNACK 2

Sandwich made with 2 slices of multigrain bread, 1 tablespoon of fat-free Miracle Whip, 1 tablespoon of sweet pickle relish, and 1 can of tuna (drained)

CALORIES: 351; PROTEIN: 44 G; FAT: 7 G; CARBS: 28 G

DINNER

1 serving of Chicken-and-Vegetable Stir-Fry

CALORIES: 314; PROTEIN: 40 G; FAT: 10 G; CARBS: 16 G

CHICKEN-AND-VEGETABLE STIR-FRY

SERVES 4

1 tablespoon canola oil

6 boneless, skinless chicken breasts, sliced into strips

1 pound frozen stir-fry vegetables

2 teaspoons fresh ginger, crushed

1 teaspoon minced garlic

¼ cup water

2 tablespoons soy sauce

Heat the oil in a large skillet or wok over high heat. Add the chicken and cook, stirring constantly, for 30 seconds, or until no longer pink on the surface. Add the vegetables, ginger, and garlic. Cook, stirring constantly, for 2 minutes, or until the vegetables are almost tender. Add the water and soy sauce. Cover, and steam for 3 minutes, or until the chicken is cooked through and the vegetables are tender-crisp.

MENU: DAY 2

BREAKFAST

1 multigrain waffle with 1 tablespoon of lite syrup

3 links of turkey sausage

1 cup of 1% cottage cheese

1 cup of 1% milk

CALORIES: 574; PROTEIN: 57 G; FAT: 22 G; CARBS: 37 G

SNACK 1

1 ounce of dry-roasted peanuts

½ cup of pineapple chunks

1 cup of 1% cottage cheese

CALORIES: 381; PROTEIN: 35 G; FAT: 17 G; CARBS: 22 G

LUNCH

Sandwich made with 2 slices of multigrain bread, 1 tablespoon of fat-free Miracle Whip, 6 ounces of fat-free turkey lunchmeat, ½ cup of spinach, and 2 slices of tomato

CALORIES: 279; PROTEIN: 30 G; FAT: 3 G; CARBS: 33 G

SNACK 2

Sandwich made with 2 slices of multigrain bread, 1 tablespoon of fat-free Miracle Whip, 1 tablespoon of sweet pickle relish, and 1 can of tuna (drained)

CALORIES: 351; PROTEIN: 44 G; FAT: 7 G; CARBS: 28 G

DINNER

1 serving of Penne with Italian Sausage and Spinach

CALORIES: 397; PROTEIN: 29 G; FAT: 17 G; CARBS: 32 G

PENNE WITH ITALIAN SAUSAGE AND SPINACH

SERVES 4

1 cup dried penne

1 pound turkey Italian sausage, cut into ¼- to ½-inch slices

1 white onion, chopped

2 teaspoons minced garlic

1 28-ounce can diced tomatoes

1 tablespoon pesto

2 cups spinach, roughly chopped

2 ounces feta cheese, crumbled

Preheat the oven to 350°F.

Cook the pasta according to the package directions. Drain, and pour into a 2-quart baking dish.

In a large skillet over medium heat, cook the sausage, onion, and garlic for 10 minutes, or until brown. Reduce the heat to medium-low. Add the tomatoes (with juice) and cook for 20 minutes. Remove from the heat. Add the pesto. Transfer to the baking dish. Stir in the spinach and cheese. Bake for 20 to 25 minutes, or until the cheese starts to bubble.

MENU: DAY 3

BREAKFAST

¾ cup of Egg Beaters or egg substitute scrambled with ⅓ cup (3 ounces) of shredded low-fat Cheddar cheese

½ cup of cantaloupe chunks

CALORIES: 254; PROTEIN: 39 G; FAT: 6 G; CARBS: 11 G

SNACK 1

1 cup of 1% cottage cheese

½ cup of pineapple chunks

CALORIES: 203; PROTEIN: 28 G; FAT: 3 G; CARBS: 16 G

LUNCH

Sandwich made with 2 slices of multigrain bread, 1 tablespoon of fat-free Miracle Whip, 1 tablespoon of sweet pickle relish, and 1 can of tuna (drained)

CALORIES: 351; PROTEIN: 44 G; FAT: 7 G; CARBS: 28 G

SNACK 2

1 piece of string cheese

1 cup of 2% chocolate milk

CALORIES: 343; PROTEIN: 24 G; FAT: 15 G; CARBS: 28 G

DINNER

1 serving of Grilled Steak

½ cup of mixed vegetables

1 multigrain roll

CALORIES: 787; PROTEIN: 53 G; FAT: 43 G; CARBS: 47 G

GRILLED STEAK

SERVES 4

4 8-ounce T-bone steaks, trimmed

Coat the grill rack with nonstick spray. Preheat the grill. Place the steaks on the prepared rack and cook, turning once, until a thermometer inserted in the center registers 145°F for medium-rare, about 10 minutes; 160°F for medium, about 12 minutes; or 165°F for well-done, about 14 minutes.

MENU: DAY 4

BREAKFAST

½ cup of rolled oats with ¼ cup of 1% milk and 1 teaspoon of brown sugar

4 links of turkey sausage

CALORIES: 462; PROTEIN: 33 G; FAT: 22 G; CARBS: 33 G

SNACK 1

1½ cups of 1% cottage cheese

1 peach

CALORIES: 284; PROTEIN: 43 G; FAT: 4 G; CARBS: 19 G

LUNCH

2 sandwiches, each made with 2 slices of multigrain bread, 1 tablespoon of fat-free Miracle Whip, 3 ounces of fat-free turkey lunchmeat, ½ cup of spinach, and 2 slices of tomato

CALORIES: 417; PROTEIN: 35 G; FAT: 5 G; CARBS: 58 G

SNACK 2

1½ cups of 1% cottage cheese

1 cup of 1% milk

CALORIES: 338; PROTEIN: 50 G; FAT: 6 G; CARBS: 21 G

DINNER

1 serving of Roasted Salmon with Goat Cheese

½ cup of green beans

CALORIES: 484; PROTEIN: 41 G; FAT: 32 G; CARBS: 8 G

ROASTED SALMON WITH GOAT CHEESE

SERVES 4

4 6- to 7-ounce salmon fillets

2 tablespoons olive oil

1 tablespoon lemon juice

¼ teaspoon salt

¼ teaspoon ground black pepper

1 clove garlic, crushed

4 ounces goat cheese, at room temperature

1 tablespoon Italian seasoning

In a baking dish, combine the oil, lemon juice, salt, pepper, and garlic. Add the fish, coat well, cover, and refrigerate for 15 minutes to 2 hours.

Meanwhile, preheat the oven to 450°F. Line a baking sheet with foil and coat it with cooking spray. Remove the fish from the marinade. Discard the marinade. Place the fish skin side down on the prepared baking sheet. Cook for 9 to 12 minutes, or until opaque. Remove from the oven and discard the skins.

In a small bowl, combine the goat cheese and the Italian seasoning. Place 2 tablespoons of the cheese mixture on top of each fillet.

BREAKFAST

¾ cup of scrambled, fried, or poached Egg Beaters or egg substitute

2 links of turkey sausage

1 slice of low-fat Cheddar cheese

2 slices of multigrain toast

CALORIES: 368; PROTEIN: 41 G; FAT: 12 G; CARBS: 24 G

SNACK 1

1 cup of 1% cottage cheese

½ cup of pineapple chunks

CALORIES: 203; PROTEIN: 28 G; FAT: 3 G; CARBS: 16 G

LUNCH

Sandwich made with 2 slices of multigrain bread, 1 tablespoon of fat-free Miracle Whip, 1 tablespoon of sweet pickle relish, and 1 can of tuna (drained)

CALORIES: 351; PROTEIN: 44 G; FAT: 7 G; CARBS: 28 G

SNACK 2

1 ounce of dry-roasted peanuts

1 cup of 1% cottage cheese

1 cup of 2% chocolate milk

CALORIES: 513; PROTEIN: 43 G; FAT: 21 G; CARBS: 38 G

DINNER

1½ servings of Chili

6 saltines

2 dill pickle spears

CALORIES: 587; PROTEIN: 51 G; FAT: 19 G; CARBS: 53 G

CHILI
SERVES 4

1 pound 90%-lean ground beef

½ cup water

1 package chili seasoning

1 16-ounce can diced tomatoes

1 can (15 ounces) kidney beans

1 can (8 ounces) tomato juice

In a large skillet over medium-high heat, cook the ground beef for 3 to 4 minutes, or until no longer pink. Drain the fat. Raise the heat to high and stir in the water, chili seasoning, tomatoes (with juice), beans (with liquid), and tomato juice. Heat to boiling. Reduce heat to low, cover, and cook for 20 minutes.

MENU: DAY 6

BREAKFAST

1 multigrain waffle with 1 tablespoon of lite syrup

3 links of turkey sausage

1 cup of 1% cottage cheese

1 cup of 1% milk

CALORIES: 574; PROTEIN: 57 G; FAT: 22 G; CARBS: 37 G

SNACK 1

1 cup of 1% milk

CALORIES: 102; PROTEIN: 8 G; FAT: 3 G; CARBS: 12 G

LUNCH

2 sandwiches, each made with 2 slices of multigrain bread, 1 tablespoon of fat-free Miracle Whip, 3 ounces of fat-free turkey lunchmeat, ½ cup of spinach, and 2 slices of tomato

CALORIES: 417; PROTEIN: 35 G; FAT: 5 G; CARBS: 58 G

SNACK 2

1½ cups of 1% cottage cheese

1 peach

CALORIES: 284; PROTEIN: 43 G; FAT: 4 G; CARBS: 19 G

DINNER

1 serving of Hamburgers

CALORIES: 540; PROTEIN: 53 G; FAT: 24 G; CARBS: 28 G

HAMBURGERS

SERVES 4

2 pounds 90%-lean ground beef

4 multigrain rolls

4 teaspoons ketchup

4 teaspoons mustard

8 slices dill pickle

1 large tomato, cut into 4 slices

Coat a grill rack or broiler pan with nonstick spray. Preheat the grill or broiler. Form the meat into 4 patties and place on the prepared rack or pan. Cook for 10 to 12 minutes, turning once, until a thermometer inserted in the center registers 160°F and the meat is no longer pink. Spread each roll with 1 teaspoon of the ketchup and 1 teaspoon of the mustard. Place 1 patty on each roll and garnish each with 2 slices of pickle and 1 slice of the tomato.

MENU: DAY 7

BREAKFAST

1   cup of Shredded
    Wheat and Bran
    with ¾ cup of
    1% milk

5   links of turkey
    sausage

CALORIES: 590; PROTEIN:
43 G; FAT: 26 G; CARBS: 46 G

SNACK 1

1½ cups of 1% cottage
    cheese

½   cup of pineapple
    chunks

CALORIES: 280; PROTEIN:
42 G; FAT: 4 G; CARBS: 19 G

LUNCH

Sandwich made
with 2 slices
of multigrain bread,
1 tablespoon of fat-
free Miracle Whip,
1 tablespoon of
sweet pickle relish,
and 1 can of tuna
(drained)

CALORIES: 351; PROTEIN:
44 G; FAT: 7 G; CARBS: 28 G

SNACK 2

1   cup of fruit
    yogurt

CALORIES: 218; PROTEIN:
9 G; FAT: 2 G; CARBS: 41 G

DINNER

2   servings of Broiled
    Shrimp Scampi

3–5 spears (¼ pound) of
    boiled or steamed
    asparagus

CALORIES: 475; PROTEIN:
41 G; FAT: 31 G; CARBS: 8 G

BROILED SHRIMP SCAMPI

SERVES 4

1   pound raw shrimp, peeled
    and deveined

¼   cup olive oil

2   teaspoons minced garlic

2   teaspoons lemon juice

¼   teaspoon salt

¼   teaspoon ground
    black pepper

2   tablespoons grated
    Parmesan cheese

Preheat the broiler. Rinse the shrimp and pat dry. In a small bowl, mix
together the oil, garlic, lemon juice, salt, and pepper. Toss the shrimp
in the oil mixture and place on the baking sheet. Sprinkle with the
cheese. Cook for 6 to 8 minutes, or until the shrimp is opaque (watch
carefully). Serve immediately.

Eating on the Fly

Those of us in the health-advice business sometimes get drunk with our own power. For example, we tell you to do things like ride a bike to work instead of driving. So let's see: You add an hour to your daily round-trip commute, fill your lungs with exhaust fumes, then have the pleasure of greeting your co-workers looking like you just bathed in canola oil—yeah, *that's* useful advice.

Telling you to swear off fast food and restaurant meals pretty much falls into the same category. Sure, these places are slaughterhouses for your diet. The cheap ones load you up with salt, high-glycemic carbs, and partially hydrogenated frying fats, while the nicer places give you oversized portions that blow your diet in one mega-sitting.

Still, try shopping with your kids on a Saturday and getting home without a spin through the drive-thru. Try spending a day in your car, calling on clients from one side of the city to the other and eating all your meals out of a brown paper bag. Try telling your boss you can't have lunch with him at Chez Snail because you'd be cheating on your diet.

So instead of dispensing impractical, Nancy Reaganesque, just-say-no advice, we herewith give you some ways to make America's flab factories work for you.

GO FISH. You yourself will probably never be able to make a slab of salmon taste as good as the one prepared by a trained chef at a nice restaurant anyway, so the first rule of eating out at a place with an actual leather-sheathed menu is this: If it has fins, it wins. Just make sure the fish is grilled, and avoid cream sauces. (On the other hand, if the menu consists of a sign above the cash registers, pass on the fish—it's fried in soybean or corn oil.)

SAY "PASTA LA VISTA." One of the authors of this book made the mistake of going to an Italian chain restaurant on his wedding night. It was a low-key wedding—just a few family members and a guy with a funny collar—and the dinner seemed like a nice way to celebrate.

That is, until he got home and fell asleep. Before . . . you know.

So excuse us if we maintain a healthy skepticism about the benefits of pasta. Not only will a serotonin-releasing starch-based meal turn your brain (and other parts) into overcooked linguine but also it will probably consist of enough food to feed most of the residents of a Calcutta alley. It comes in a big bowl, and you can eat and eat and eat and not feel full until a few minutes before you pass out.

More to the point, pasta-based dishes don't serve you well on the T diet. It's theoretically possible to balance the protein, carbs, and fat if it's a pasta dish laced with fish or meat, but you have to leave most of the noodles in the bowl. It's easier to just pass over this portion of the menu altogether.

SANDBAG SANDWICHES. Sub shops are great places to load up on protein. A 6-inch roasted chicken breast sandwich at Subway contains 25 grams of protein, about one-third of the total calories. But it's tough to keep a balance of fat and carbs. And if you balance those two macronutrients, as in a 6-inch Subway Southwest Steak and Cheese, you come out light on protein (only about 22 percent of total calories).

Tuna-salad sandwiches are surprisingly poor choices: They're made with mayonnaise, which is filled with trans fats. Plus, they usually have less protein than the meat sandwiches.

Your best bets in sub shops tend to be chicken and turkey on whole grain bread. Make sure the chicken is grilled, not breaded—you don't need the extra carbs. Go heavy on the green peppers, black olives, lettuce, pickles, tomatoes, and onions. These add flavor, texture, and nutrients to the sandwich without piling on many extra calories.

When given a choice of condiments, choose oil and vinegar over mayo. (Ask what type of oil is used; Subway uses canola oil and extra virgin olive oil.) Even with the oil, you probably won't be able to balance the carbohydrates in the bread. No biggie—just cut a few carbs later in the day.

DOWNSIZE. A Big Mac, large fries, and medium Coke at McDonald's deliver more than 1,300 calories. Supersize it, and you're over 1,600 calories. For one meal. Never mind the balance of fat, carbs, and protein—you're drowning in calories before the protein has a chance to do its work.

Your goal is to get out of there with 500 to 700 calories in your stomach, including a balance of fat and carbohydrate. See the bottom of pages 128 and 129 for four ways to do it, with one caveat: Most of the fat in these meals is saturated, most of the carbs are in the

(continued)

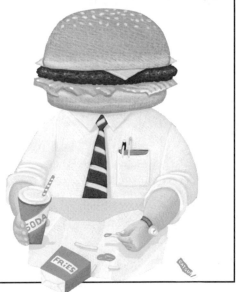

form of white bread, and the food is saltier than the Bonneville flats. When you eat stuff like this, make sure the day's other meals have as little saturated fat, high-glycemic carbs, and salt as possible.

Be aware that these are *general* guidelines for the hypothetical average reader; it's impossible for us to tweak a fast-food conglomerate's long-established menu with an eye toward the special, individualized goals of every possible reader on each version of our plan. So we're not going to tell you that if you weigh 230 pounds and are looking to lose flab, you should eat only five-eighths of a Big Mac or 83.4 percent of your hash browns. Regardless of your current weight or your goals, just try to stay somewhere within these guidelines—and realize that you shouldn't be doing very much of your eating in fast-food restaurants in the first place.

SHOULD YOU PAN PIZZA? We checked three different types of Pizza Hut crusts—thin, stuffed, and hand-tossed—and found that the fat and carbohydrate calories come out about even. The only problem for T-dieters is that the protein is fairly low. For example, if you have two slices of Pizza Hut stuffed-crust pepperoni pizza, you're getting 346 calories from fat, 360 from carbs, and just 168 from protein. That ratio kinda sorta works for a skinny guy trying to gain weight: It's about 19 percent protein, 41 percent carbs, and 40 percent fat. But it's light on protein for guys trying to maintain or lose weight.

Another issue is that about half the fat is saturated: You take in a day's worth with just two slices.

If you have pizza at one meal while trying to gain or maintain weight, make sure you increase protein later in the day. Whatever your body-composition goal, you should definitely avoid saturated fat in your other meals.

DROP THE CHALUPA. It's not hard to

McDONALD'S BREAKFAST

2 Egg McMuffins

CALORIES: 580; PROTEIN: 34 G
(ABOUT 23 PERCENT OF CALORIES);
FAT: 24 G (ABOUT 37 PERCENT OF
CALORIES); CARBOHYDRATE: 54 G
(ABOUT 37 PERCENT OF CALORIES)

McDONALD'S LUNCH OR DINNER

Quarter Pounder
Reduced-fat vanilla ice cream cone

CALORIES: 580; PROTEIN: 27 G
(ABOUT 19 PERCENT OF CALORIES);
FAT: 25.5 G (ABOUT 40 PERCENT OF
CALORIES); CARBOHYDRATE: 60 G
(ABOUT 42 PERCENT OF CALORIES)

get a balance of protein, fat, and carbs at pseudo-Mexican chains like Taco Bell and Del Taco. (Real Mexicans don't eat this stuff, just so you know.) For example, the steak soft taco at Taco Bell has 30 percent protein, with 32 percent fat and 38 percent carbs. The drawback is the 980 milligrams of sodium in two steak tacos. That's close to half a day's worth, figuring the average guy should take in about 2,400 milligrams.

Skip anything deep-fried or double-decked. And substitute guacamole for sour cream—both toppings are mostly fat, but the fat in the avocado-rich guacamole is monounsaturated.

Taco salads can also be decent choices, especially if salsa is used as the dressing.

SCRUTINIZE CHINESE. Remember the good old days, when hack comedians made jokes that were not-so-sly allusions to the fact that you could fill up on Chinese food and be hungry an hour later? (Typical line: "I just picked up my clothes at the Chinese laundry an hour ago—and now they feel dirty again." Ba-dump-bump.) That's because Chinese food, as a rule, was high in carbohydrate, very low in protein, and somewhat low in fat.

Today, we're happy to report that Chinese food is soaked in fat. For example, according to a 1994 study by the Center for Science in the Public Interest, a typical dinner-size order of Kung Pao chicken has 76 grams of fat. Most of the fat comes from peanuts, which means it's mostly monounsaturated. The study didn't go into detail about protein and carbs, although they did say most of the Chinese dishes they studied were overloaded with salt.

Our recommendation is that you stick with dishes heavy in meat and nuts: cashew chicken, beef with broccoli, Szechuan shrimp, or shrimp with garlic sauce. And go light on the white rice; it can turn an otherwise hearty, protein-rich meal into a sleep-inducing carb fest.

BURGER KING LUNCH OR DINNER

Chicken club sandwich (no mayo)

CALORIES: 530; PROTEIN: 30 G (ABOUT 23 PERCENT OF CALORIES); FAT: 21 G (ABOUT 36 PERCENT OF CALORIES); CARBOHYDRATE: 54 G (ABOUT 41 PERCENT OF CALORIES)

WENDY'S LUNCH OR DINNER

Large chili

Classic Single

CALORIES: 670; PROTEIN: 47 G (ABOUT 28 PERCENT OF CALORIES); FAT: 26 G (ABOUT 35 PERCENT OF CALORIES); CARBOHYDRATE: 63 G (ABOUT 40 PERCENT OF CALORIES)

CRUISERWEIGHT

GROCERY LIST

ONE-TIME ITEMS

Olive oil
Canola oil
Dry-roasted peanuts
Soy sauce
Minced garlic
Ketchup
Mustard

Dill pickles
Sweet pickle relish
Brown sugar
Fresh ginger
Italian seasoning
Salt
Ground black pepper

Lemon juice
Dijon mustard
Mayonnaise
Peanut butter
Jelly
Lite syrup

WEEKLY ITEMS

1½ gallons of 1% milk
2 quarts of 2% chocolate milk
1 quart of apple juice
1 cup of orange juice
1 12-ounce container of 1% cottage cheese
1 16-ounce bag of shredded low-fat Cheddar cheese
1 16-ounce bag of shredded mozzarella cheese
1 package of Cheddar cheese slices
1 small block of Parmesan cheese
3 ounces of feta cheese
4 ounces of goat cheese
1 small container of cream cheese
2 containers of full-fat fruit yogurt
1 dozen large eggs
3 6-ounce cans of water-packed tuna
2 loaves of thin multigrain bread

8 multigrain rolls
2 plain bagels
½ pound of spinach
5 tomatoes
1 white onion
1 pound of asparagus
1 cantaloupe
1 pineapple or 1 cup of pineapple chunks
3 oranges
1 banana
1 1-pound bag of frozen stir-fry vegetables
1 pound of green beans
1 1-pound bag of frozen mixed vegetables
1 box of multigrain waffles
1 pound of turkey Italian sausage
2 packages of turkey sausage links
1½ pounds of boneless, skinless chicken breasts
1¼ pounds of roasted or smoked turkey lunchmeat

½ pound of sliced ham
1 pound of bacon
4 6- to 7-ounce salmon fillets
1 pound of raw shrimp
2 pounds of T-bone steak
3 pounds of at least 90%-lean ground beef
1 container of pesto
1 box of dried penne
1 box of brown rice
1 box of rolled oats
1 box of Shredded Wheat and Bran
1 package of chili seasoning
1 15-ounce can of kidney beans
1 8-ounce can of tomato juice
1 28-ounce and 1 16-ounce can of diced tomatoes
1 12-ounce can of barbecue baked beans
1 box of saltines
1 box of granola

BREAKFAST

1¾ cups of Shredded Wheat and Bran with 1 cup of 1% milk

3 links of turkey breakfast sausage

½ cup of pineapple chunks

CALORIES: 658; PROTEIN: 37 G; FAT: 18 G; CARBS: 87 G

SNACK 1

2 ounces of dry-roasted peanuts

1 cup of 1% milk

CALORIES: 459; PROTEIN: 21 G; FAT: 31 G; CARBS: 24 G

LUNCH

2 sandwiches, each made with 2 slices of multigrain bread, 1 tablespoon of mayonnaise, 3 ounces of turkey lunchmeat, ¼ cup of spinach, and 2 slices of tomato

1 medium orange

CALORIES: 676; PROTEIN: 38 G; FAT: 28 G; CARBS: 68 G

SNACK 2

1 ounce of dry-roasted peanuts

1 cup of 2% chocolate milk

CALORIES: 359; PROTEIN: 15 G; FAT: 19 G; CARBS: 32 G

DINNER

1 serving of Chicken-and-Vegetable Stir-Fry

CALORIES: 586; PROTEIN: 44 G; FAT: 22 G; CARBS: 53 G

CHICKEN-AND-VEGETABLE STIR-FRY

SERVES 4

1 cup brown rice

¼ cup canola oil

6 boneless, skinless chicken breasts, sliced into strips

1 pound frozen stir-fry vegetables

2 teaspoons fresh ginger, crushed

1 teaspoon minced garlic

¼ cup water

2 tablespoons soy sauce

Cook the rice according to the package directions. Keep warm. Heat the oil in a large skillet or wok over high heat. Add the chicken and cook, stirring constantly, for 30 seconds, or until no longer pink on the surface. Add the vegetables, ginger, and garlic. Cook, stirring constantly, for 2 minutes, or until the vegetables are almost tender. Add the water and soy sauce. Cover, and steam for 3 minutes, or until the chicken is cooked through and the vegetables are tender-crisp. Serve over the rice.

BREAKFAST

3 multigrain waffles with 3 tablespoons of lite syrup

3 links of turkey sausage

1 cup of 1% milk

CALORIES: 646; PROTEIN: 34 G; FAT: 26 G; CARBS: 69 G

SNACK 1

1 ounce of dry-roasted peanuts

½ cup of 1% cottage cheese

1 cup of 2% chocolate milk

CALORIES: 436; PROTEIN: 29 G; FAT: 20 G; CARBS: 35 G

LUNCH

2 sandwiches, each made with 2 slices of multigrain bread, 1 tablespoon of mayonnaise, 1 tablespoon of Dijon mustard, 2 ounces of turkey lunchmeat, ½ cup of spinach, and 2 slices of tomato

1 cup of apple juice

CALORIES: 683; PROTEIN: 31 G; FAT: 27 G; CARBS: 79 G

SNACK 2

1 ounce of dry-roasted peanuts

1 cup of 2% chocolate milk

CALORIES: 359; PROTEIN: 15 G; FAT: 19 G; CARBS: 32 G

DINNER

1 serving of Penne with Italian Sausage and Spinach

CALORIES: 616; PROTEIN: 40 G; FAT: 28 G; CARBS: 51 G

PENNE WITH ITALIAN SAUSAGE AND SPINACH

SERVES 4

2 cups dried penne

1 pound turkey Italian sausage, cut into ¼- to ½-inch slices

1 white onion, chopped

2 teaspoons minced garlic

1 28-ounce can diced tomatoes

¼ cup pesto

2 cups spinach, roughly chopped

3 ounces feta cheese, crumbled

⅓ cup shredded mozzarella cheese

Preheat the oven to 350°F.

Cook the pasta according to the package directions. Drain, and pour into a 2-quart baking dish.

In a large skillet over medium heat, cook the sausage, onion, and garlic for 10 minutes, or until brown. Reduce the heat to medium-low. Add the tomatoes (with juice) and cook for 20 minutes. Remove the skillet from the heat. Add the pesto. Transfer to the baking dish. Stir in the spinach and feta cheese. Sprinkle with the mozzarella. Bake for 20 to 25 minutes, or until the cheese starts to bubble.

MENU: DAY 3

BREAKFAST

2 large eggs scrambled with ⅓ cup of shredded Cheddar cheese

2 slices of ham

2 slices of multigrain toast, each with 1 tablespoon of jelly

½ cup of cantaloupe chunks

CALORIES: 664; PROTEIN: 36 G; FAT: 32 G; CARBS: 58 G

SNACK 1

1 ounce of dry-roasted peanuts

1 cup of apple juice

CALORIES: 298; PROTEIN: 8 G; FAT: 14 G; CARBS: 35 G

LUNCH

2 sandwiches, each made with 2 slices of multigrain bread, ½ tablespoon of mayonnaise, ½ tablespoon of sweet pickle relish, and ½ can of tuna (drained)

1 medium orange

CALORIES: 610; PROTEIN: 50 G; FAT: 18 G; CARBS: 62 G

SNACK 2

1 plain bagel with 1 tablespoon of cream cheese

CALORIES: 351; PROTEIN: 13 G; FAT: 7 G; CARBS: 59 G

DINNER

1 serving of Grilled Steak

½ cup of mixed vegetables

1 multigrain roll

CALORIES: 787; PROTEIN: 53 G; FAT: 43 G; CARBS: 47 G

GRILLED STEAK

SERVES 4

4 8-ounce T-bone steaks, trimmed

Coat the grill rack with nonstick spray. Preheat the grill. Place the steaks on the prepared rack and cook, turning once, until a thermometer inserted in the center registers 145°F for medium-rare, about 10 minutes; 160°F for medium, about 12 minutes; or 165°F for well-done, about 14 minutes.

MENU: DAY 4

BREAKFAST

1 cup of rolled oats with ¼ cup of 1% milk and 1 teaspoon of brown sugar

2 links of turkey sausage

1 slice of multigrain toast with 1 tablespoon of jelly

1 cup of orange juice

CALORIES: 692; PROTEIN: 30 G; FAT: 16 G; CARBS: 107 G

SNACK 1

1 ounce of dry-roasted peanuts

1 cup of 1% cottage cheese

CALORIES: 332; PROTEIN: 35 G; FAT: 16 G; CARBS: 12 G

LUNCH

2 sandwiches, each made with 2 slices of multigrain bread, 1 tablespoon of mayonnaise, 3 ounces of turkey lunchmeat, ½ cup of spinach, and 2 slices of tomato

1 medium orange

CALORIES: 684; PROTEIN: 40 G; FAT: 28 G; CARBS: 68 G

SNACK 2

1 ounce of dry-roasted peanuts

1 cup of 2% chocolate milk

CALORIES: 359; PROTEIN: 15 G; FAT: 19 G; CARBS: 32 G

DINNER

1 serving of Roasted Salmon with Goat Cheese

½ cup of green beans

1 multigrain roll

CALORIES: 676; PROTEIN: 48 G; FAT: 36 G; CARBS: 40 G

ROASTED SALMON WITH GOAT CHEESE

SERVES 4

4 6- to 7-ounce salmon fillets

2 tablespoons olive oil

1 tablespoon lemon juice

¼ teaspoon salt

¼ teaspoon ground black pepper

1 clove garlic, crushed

4 ounces goat cheese, at room temperature

1 tablespoon Italian seasoning

In a baking dish, combine the oil, lemon juice, salt, pepper, and garlic. Add the fish, coat well, cover, and refrigerate for 15 minutes to 2 hours. Meanwhile, preheat the oven to 450°F. Line a baking sheet with foil and coat it with cooking spray.

Remove the fish from the marinade. Discard the marinade. Place the fish skin side down on the prepared baking sheet. Cook for 9 to 12 minutes, or until opaque. Remove from the oven and discard the skins. In a small bowl, combine the goat cheese and the Italian seasoning. Place 2 tablespoons of the cheese mixture on top of each fillet.

BREAKFAST

1 large egg, scrambled or poached

2 strips of bacon

1 slice of Cheddar cheese

2 slices of multigrain toast, each with 1 tablespoon of jelly

CALORIES: 613; PROTEIN: 29 G; FAT: 33 G; CARBS: 50 G

SNACK 1

1 cup of fruit yogurt

1 cup of apple juice

CALORIES: 338; PROTEIN: 10 G; FAT: 2 G; CARBS: 70 G

LUNCH

2 sandwiches, each made with 2 slices of multigrain bread, ½ tablespoon of mayonnaise, ½ tablespoon of sweet pickle relish, and ½ can of tuna (drained)

1 medium orange

CALORIES: 610; PROTEIN: 50 G; FAT: 18 G; CARBS: 62 G

SNACK 2

2 ounces of dry-roasted peanuts

1 cup of 2% chocolate milk

CALORIES: 533; PROTEIN: 21 G; FAT: 33 G; CARBS: 38 G

DINNER

1½ servings of Chili

6 saltines

2 dill pickle spears

CALORIES: 587; PROTEIN: 51 G; FAT: 19 G; CARBS: 53 G

CHILI

SERVES 4

1 pound 90%-lean ground beef

½ cup water

1 package chili seasoning

1 16-ounce can diced tomatoes

1 can (15 ounces) kidney beans

1 can (8 ounces) tomato juice

In a large skillet over medium-high heat, cook the ground beef for 3 to 4 minutes, or until no longer pink. Drain the fat. Raise the heat to high and stir in the water, chili seasoning, tomatoes (with juice), beans (with liquid), and tomato juice. Heat to boiling. Reduce heat to low, cover, and cook for 20 minutes.

MENU: DAY 6

BREAKFAST

3 multigrain waffles with 3 tablespoons of lite syrup

3 links of turkey sausage

1 cup of 1% milk

CALORIES: 646; PROTEIN: 34 G; FAT: 26 G; CARBS: 69 G

SNACK 1

1 plain bagel with 2 tablespoons of peanut butter

CALORIES: 502; PROTEIN: 20 G; FAT: 18 G; CARBS: 65 G

LUNCH

Sandwich made with 2 slices of multigrain bread, 1 tablespoon of mayonnaise, 1 tablespoon of Dijon mustard, 4 ounces of turkey lunch-meat, ½ cup of spinach, and 2 slices of tomato

1 cup of apple juice

CALORIES: 454; PROTEIN: 26 G; FAT: 14 G; CARBS: 56 G

SNACK 2

2 ounces of dry-roasted peanuts

1 cup of 1% milk

CALORIES: 459; PROTEIN: 21 G; FAT: 31 G; CARBS: 24 G

DINNER

1 serving of Hamburgers

⅓ cup of barbecue baked beans

CALORIES: 657; PROTEIN: 58 G; FAT: 25 G; CARBS: 50 G

HAMBURGERS

SERVES 4

2 pounds 90%-lean ground beef

4 multigrain rolls

4 teaspoons ketchup

4 teaspoons mustard

8 slices dill pickle

1 large tomato, cut into 4 slices

Coat a grill rack or broiler pan with nonstick spray. Preheat the grill or broiler. Form the meat into 4 patties and place on the prepared rack or pan. Cook for 10 to 12 minutes, turning once, until a thermometer inserted in the center registers 160°F and the meat is no longer pink. Spread each roll with 1 teaspoon of the ketchup and 1 teaspoon of the mustard. Place 1 patty on each roll and garnish each with 2 slices of pickle and 1 slice of the tomato.

BREAKFAST

1¾ cups of Shredded Wheat and Bran with 1 cup of 1% milk

4 links of turkey sausage

½ cup of pineapple chunks

CALORIES: 727; PROTEIN: 43 G; FAT: 23 G; CARBS: 87 G

SNACK 1

1 cup of fruit yogurt

1 ounce of granola

CALORIES: 336; PROTEIN: 15 G; FAT: 6 G; CARBS: 86 G

LUNCH

2 sandwiches, each made with 2 slices of multigrain bread, ½ tablespoon of mayonnaise, ½ tablespoon of sweet pickle relish, and ½ can of tuna (drained)

1 medium orange

CALORIES: 610; PROTEIN: 50 G; FAT: 18 G; CARBS: 62 G

SNACK 2

2 ounces of dry-roasted peanuts

1 banana

CALORIES: 481; PROTEIN: 15 G; FAT: 29 G; CARBS: 40 G

DINNER

2 servings of Broiled Shrimp Scampi

3–5 spears (¼ pound) of boiled or steamed asparagus

CALORIES: 475; PROTEIN: 41 G; FAT: 31 G; CARBS: 8 G

BROILED SHRIMP SCAMPI

SERVES 4

1 pound raw shrimp, peeled and deveined

¼ cup olive oil

2 teaspoons minced garlic

2 teaspoons lemon juice

¼ teaspoon salt

¼ teaspoon ground black pepper

2 tablespoons grated Parmesan cheese

Preheat the broiler. Rinse the shrimp and pat dry. In a small bowl, mix together the oil, garlic, lemon juice, salt, and pepper. Toss the shrimp in the oil mixture and place on the baking sheet. Sprinkle with the cheese. Cook for 6 to 8 minutes, or until the shrimp is opaque (watch carefully). Serve immediately.

Sweet Indulgences

When we first started a few dozen of our friends and co-workers on the T diet, we were a little worried about how they'd react to being told what to eat. Turns out they didn't have much of a problem with it, especially when we mentioned that meat and fat are integral parts of the plan.

It's when they saw what they *couldn't* eat that they got a little testy. No chips? No candy? And where the hell are the Little Debbies?

Look, we understand the calming effect of a bowl of cookie dough ice cream at the end of the night. We know you'll feel like a dork and look like a self-righteous nutrition Nazi if you pass up a slice of cake at your daughter's birthday party. Nobody wants to be the buzz killer who says, "No thanks, I'm on a diet. I'll just watch you guys get fat and die early."

We also know you live in a world filled with fatty, sugary, salty snacks. We live there, too. Whether you're in a grocery store, a gas station, or the company cafeteria, there's no getting away from them. And to top it all off, cocoa producers bombard consumers with research showing that chocolate contains antioxidants and other chemicals known to help ward off heart disease, cancer, and strokes.

So the last thing we're going to tell you is that you can never, ever indulge for the rest of your life. Instead, we're going to suggest some strategies to help you pick your moments and limit the collateral damage.

PROTEIN FIRST, SWEETS LATER. Since protein is the macronutrient that makes you feel fullest, if you save your sweets for the end of a protein-rich meal, it stands to reason that you'll eat fewer of them. And the converse is also true. Sweets are filled with sugar and fat, neither of which makes you feel satiated during a meal. Eat them on an empty stomach, and you can inhale 1,000 calories of carbohydrate and fat faster than we can type the words advising you not to.

Next time you hear the siren call of the cookie dough ice cream, try this: Eat a peanut butter and jelly sandwich on whole grain bread. Chase it with a glass of 1% or 2% milk. If you still hear the cookie dough calling—even with some protein, fat, and carbs in your stomach—go ahead and answer. Just remember to . . .

PAY ATTENTION TO HOW MUCH YOU'RE EATING. Recently, one of our co-authors bought a new set of dishes. He likes them—they're heavy and manly and durable—but when he opened the box they came in, the first thing he noticed is that the bowls are big enough to mix cement in. Thus what looks like a single serving is actually enough to feed a championship sumo wrestler.

So he resorted to a strategy that we recommend for you: Measure sweets before you eat them. Grab a measuring cup, spoon out exactly 1 cup of ice cream, put it in the bowl, and enjoy it.

This technique works with any type of dessert. Look on the package and see what's considered a serving. Measure it out. Eat it slowly, enjoying each bite.

Still want more? Fine. All we ask is that you . . .

WAIT 20 MINUTES BETWEEN SERVINGS. This is the nutritional equivalent of the half-hour background check that a gun shop does before it sends someone out with a 9 millimeter. Twenty minutes is usually enough time for your body to notice that you've eaten. And just as that half-hour background check will hopefully identify anyone who shouldn't be in possession of a firearm, so too will your culinary cooling-off period help you realize that you really don't need a second helping of your kid's birthday cake.

And birthday cake is a pretty good example of the next rule of indulgence, which says . . .

IF YOU'RE GOING TO CHEAT, JUST CHEAT! Don't eat something that isn't what you really want. If your stomach is screaming for Snickers, pretzels won't stifle the noise. You'll probably wind up eating the pretzels, then running out for the Snickers later, too.

Sure, you'll feel superior if you buy an Entenmann's fat-free pound cake instead of the real thing. But you'll realize pretty quickly that it takes three or four times as much of the virtuous version to achieve the satisfaction you would've gotten from one slice of the sinful stuff.

Of course, this strategy works only if you . . .

PICK YOUR SPOTS. Be honest with yourself: At least half the time you indulge, it's out of habit, not an overwhelming desire to tear into a jelly doughnut. So you need to be selective. Say your anniversary is coming up and your wife is dropping not-so-subtle hints that she wants to go out for a big, fancy,

(continued)

expensive dinner. Since you know you're going to have dessert that night, you can pass up one or two treats in the preceding nights. When you get caught by surprise with an office birthday party, fine, have the cake. Make up for it by skipping a dessert later in the week.

Almost all the lean people we know give themselves a "cheat" meal once a week, when they can eat the things that lean people normally avoid. This strategy acknowledges that special occasions come up. But unless you have a much more interesting life than we do, they don't come up every day.

This brings us to our final point about sweets:

YOUR LEAN BODY IS A BETTER REWARD THAN A DAILY DESSERT. One of the guys who tried out the T diet at first complained that he missed his nightly bag of chips. This guy works brutally hard—he's at the office or on his laptop nearly every waking hour—and he saw the bag of chips that he ate while he watched *SportsCenter* as the one part of the day when he didn't have to be accountable to anyone.

But then he lost a chunk of weight on the T diet, rediscovered the satisfaction of a hard workout, and changed his point of view. He found that the workouts provide more stress relief than the chips did. The chips offered a reward that lasted an hour or two. The diet and workouts give him satisfaction around the clock. When he's awake, he can look in the mirror and see his younger, more vital self. At night, his sleep is deeper; and in the morning, he wakes up feeling more rested and energetic.

A Final Word on Sweets

So you broke all the rules and ate three pieces of cake. You screwed up. It's not the end of the world—or even the end of the diet. Successful weight management is about eating right *most* of the time, not all of the time. Consistency isn't the same as rigidity.

We want you to be diligent in your diet. We think the T diet makes it easier by incorporating many of the foods you already like. But it doesn't include all of them. If you need to indulge in some off-diet treats for the pure, hedonistic pleasure of it, we aren't going to be the ones to say that you're going to nutritional hell in a picnic basket. When you need a goody, get one. When you don't, give it a pass.

WELTERWEIGHT

ONE-TIME ITEMS

Olive oil

Canola oil

Dry-roasted peanuts

Soy sauce

Minced garlic

Ketchup

Mustard

Dill pickles

Sweet pickle relish

Brown sugar

Fresh ginger

Italian seasoning

Salt

Ground black pepper

Lemon juice

Dijon mustard

Mayonnaise

Peanut butter

Jelly

Butter

Lite syrup

WEEKLY ITEMS

1½ gallons of 1% milk

1 gallon of 2% chocolate milk

1 quart of apple juice

1 pint of orange juice

1 16-ounce bag of shredded Cheddar cheese

1 16-ounce bag of shredded mozzarella cheese

1 small block of Cheddar cheese slices

1 small block of Parmesan cheese

3 ounces of feta cheese

4 ounces of goat cheese

2 containers of full-fat fruit yogurt

1 dozen large eggs

2 6-ounce cans of water-packed tuna

2 loaves of thin multigrain bread

5 multigrain rolls

3 plain bagels

1¾ pounds of spinach

¼ cup of chopped walnuts

4 tomatoes

1 white onion

1 pound of asparagus

1 cantaloupe

1 pineapple or ½ cup of pineapple chunks

4 oranges

1 large apple

3 bananas

1 pint of blueberries

1 1-pound bag of frozen stir-fry vegetables

1 pound of green beans

1 1-pound bag of frozen mixed vegetables

1 box of frozen multigrain waffles

2 pounds of turkey Italian sausage

2 packages of turkey sausage links

1½ pounds of boneless, skinless chicken breasts

1¼ pounds of roasted or smoked turkey lunchmeat

½ pound of sliced ham

1 pound of bacon

4 6- to 7-ounce salmon fillets

1 pound of raw shrimp

2 pounds of T-bone steak

2½ pounds of at least 90%-lean ground beef

1 container of pesto

1 box of dried penne

1 box of brown rice

1 box of rolled oats

1 box of Shredded Wheat and Bran

1 package of chili seasoning

1 15-ounce can of kidney beans

1 8-ounce can of tomato juice

1 28-ounce and 1 16-ounce can of diced tomatoes

1 12-ounce can of barbecue baked beans

1 box of saltines

1 box of granola

MENU: DAY 1

BREAKFAST

1¾ cups Shredded Wheat and Bran with 1 cup of 1% milk

3 links of turkey breakfast sausage

½ cup of pineapple chunks

CALORIES: 658; PROTEIN: 37 G; FAT: 18 G; CARBS: 87 G

SNACK 1

1 plain bagel with 2 tablespoons of peanut butter

CALORIES: 502; PROTEIN: 20 G; FAT: 18 G; CARBS: 65 G

LUNCH

2 sandwiches, each made with 2 slices of multigrain bread, 1 tablespoon of mayonnaise, 2 ounces of turkey lunchmeat, ½ cup of spinach, and 2 slices of tomato

1 medium orange

CALORIES: 623; PROTEIN: 30 G; FAT: 27 G; CARBS: 65 G

SNACK 2

2 ounces of dry-roasted peanuts

1 cup of 1% milk

CALORIES: 463; PROTEIN: 22 G; FAT: 31 G; CARBS: 24 G

DINNER

1 serving of Chicken-and-Vegetable Stir-Fry

CALORIES: 759; PROTEIN: 37 G; FAT: 27 G; CARBS: 92 G

CHICKEN-AND-VEGETABLE STIR-FRY

SERVES 4

2 cups brown rice

¼ cup canola oil

4 boneless, skinless chicken breasts, sliced into strips

1 pound frozen stir-fry vegetables

2 teaspoons fresh ginger, crushed

1 teaspoon minced garlic

¼ cup water

2 tablespoons soy sauce

¼ cup chopped walnut pieces

Cook the rice according to the package directions. Keep warm. Heat the oil in a large skillet or wok over high heat. Add the chicken and cook, stirring constantly, for 30 seconds, or until no longer pink on the surface. Add the vegetables, ginger, and garlic. Cook, stirring constantly, for 2 minutes, or until the vegetables are almost tender. Add the water and soy sauce. Cover, and steam for 3 minutes, or until the chicken is cooked through and the vegetables are tender-crisp. Stir in the walnuts and serve over the rice.

MENU: DAY 2

BREAKFAST

5 multigrain waffles with 5 tablespoons of lite syrup

3 strips of bacon

1 cup of 1% milk

CALORIES: 775; PROTEIN: 26 G; FAT: 27 G; CARBS: 107 G

SNACK 1

2 ounces of dry-roasted peanuts

1 cup of 2% chocolate milk

CALORIES: 533; PROTEIN: 21 G; FAT: 33 G; CARBS: 38 G

LUNCH

2 sandwiches, each made with 2 slices of multigrain bread, 1 tablespoon of mayonnaise, 3 ounces of turkey lunchmeat, ½ cup of spinach, and 2 slices of tomato

CALORIES: 616; PROTEIN: 39 G; FAT: 28 G; CARBS: 52 G

SNACK 2

2 ounces of dry-roasted peanuts

1 cup of apple juice

CALORIES: 472; PROTEIN: 14 G; FAT: 28 G; CARBS: 41 G

DINNER

1 serving of Penne with Italian Sausage and Spinach

CALORIES: 616; PROTEIN: 40 G; FAT: 28 G; CARBS: 51 G

PENNE WITH ITALIAN SAUSAGE AND SPINACH

SERVES 4

2 cups dried penne

1 pound turkey Italian sausage, cut into ¼- to ½-inch slices

1 white onion, chopped

2 teaspoons minced garlic

1 28-ounce can diced tomatoes

¼ cup pesto

2 cups spinach, roughly chopped

3 ounces feta cheese, crumbled

⅓ cup shredded mozzarella cheese

Preheat the oven to 350°F.

Cook the pasta according to the package directions. Drain, and pour into a 2-quart baking dish.

In a large skillet over medium heat, cook the sausage, onion, and garlic for 10 minutes, or until brown. Reduce the heat to medium-low. Add the tomatoes (with juice) and cook for 20 minutes. Remove the skillet from the heat. Add the pesto. Transfer to the baking dish. Stir in the spinach and feta cheese. Sprinkle with the mozzarella. Bake for 20 to 25 minutes, or until the cheese starts to bubble.

BREAKFAST

2 large eggs scrambled
  with ⅓ cup of
  shredded Cheddar
  cheese

2 slices of ham

2 slices of multigrain
  toast, each with 1
  tablespoon of jelly

½ cup of cantaloupe
  chunks

CALORIES: 664; PROTEIN:
36 G; FAT: 32 G; CARBS: 58 G

SNACK 1

1 ounce of dry-
  roasted peanuts

1 cup of fruit yogurt

1 cup of apple juice

CALORIES: 516; PROTEIN:
17 G; FAT: 16 G; CARBS: 76 G

LUNCH

Sandwich made
with 2 slices of
multigrain bread,
1 tablespoon of
mayonnaise,
1 tablespoon of
sweet pickle relish,
and ½ can of tuna
(drained)

1 medium orange

CALORIES: 399; PROTEIN:
25 G; FAT: 15 G; CARBS: 41 G

SNACK 2

1 plain bagel with
  2 tablespoons of
  peanut butter and
  2 tablespoons of
  jelly

CALORIES: 610; PROTEIN:
20 G; FAT: 18 G; CARBS: 92 G

DINNER

1 serving of Grilled
  Steak

½ cup of mixed
  vegetables

1 multigrain roll

CALORIES: 787; PROTEIN:
53 G; FAT: 43 G; CARBS: 47 G

GRILLED STEAK

SERVES 4

4 8-ounce T-bone steaks,
  trimmed

Coat the grill rack with nonstick spray. Preheat the grill. Place the
steaks on the prepared rack and cook, turning once, until a thermometer inserted in the center registers 145°F for medium-rare, about
10 minutes; 160°F for medium, about 12 minutes; or 165°F for well-
done, about 14 minutes.

BREAKFAST

1 cup of rolled oats with ¼ cup of 1% milk and 2 teaspoons of brown sugar

2 links of turkey sausage

1 slice of multigrain toast with 1 tablespoon of jelly

1 cup of orange juice

CALORIES: 712; PROTEIN: 30 G; FAT: 16 G; CARBS: 112 G

SNACK 1

1 ounce of dry-roasted peanuts

1 cup of apple juice

CALORIES: 298; PROTEIN: 8 G; FAT: 14 G; CARBS: 35 G

LUNCH

2 sandwiches, each made with 2 slices of multigrain bread, 1 tablespoon of mayonnaise, 3 ounces of turkey lunchmeat, ½ cup of spinach, and 2 slices of tomato

1 banana

CALORIES: 724; PROTEIN: 39 G; FAT: 28 G; CARBS: 79 G

SNACK 2

2 ounces of dry-roasted peanuts

1 cup of 2% chocolate milk

CALORIES: 533; PROTEIN: 21 G; FAT: 33 G; CARBS: 38 G

DINNER

1 serving of Roasted Salmon with Goat Cheese

½ cup of green beans

1 multigrain roll with 1 tablespoon of butter

CALORIES: 784; PROTEIN: 48 G; FAT: 48 G; CARBS: 40 G

ROASTED SALMON WITH GOAT CHEESE

SERVES 4

4 6- to 7-ounce salmon fillets

2 tablespoons olive oil

1 tablespoon lemon juice

¼ teaspoon salt

¼ teaspoon ground black pepper

1 clove garlic, crushed

4 ounces goat cheese, at room temperature

1 tablespoon Italian seasoning

In a baking dish, combine the oil, lemon juice, salt, pepper, and garlic. Add the fish, coat well, cover, and refrigerate for 15 minutes to 2 hours.

Meanwhile, preheat the oven to 450°F. Line a baking sheet with foil and coat it with cooking spray.

Remove the fish from the marinade. Discard the marinade. Place the fish skin side down on the prepared baking sheet. Cook for 9 to 12 minutes, or until opaque. Remove from the oven and discard the skins. In a small bowl, combine the goat cheese and the Italian seasoning. Place 2 tablespoons of the cheese mixture on top of each fillet.

BREAKFAST

1   large egg, fried, scrambled, or poached

2   strips of bacon

1   slice of Cheddar cheese

4   slices of multigrain toast, each with ½ tablespoon of jelly

CALORIES: 609; PROTEIN: 26 G; FAT: 25 G; CARBS: 70 G

SNACK 1

2   ounces of dry-roasted peanuts

1   cup of apple juice

CALORIES: 472; PROTEIN: 14 G; FAT: 28 G; CARBS: 41 G

LUNCH

Sandwich made with 2 of slices multigrain bread, 1 tablespoon of mayonnaise, 1 tablespoon of sweet pickle relish, and ½ can of tuna (drained)

1   medium orange

1   cup of 2% chocolate milk

CALORIES: 584; PROTEIN: 34 G; FAT: 20 G; CARBS: 67 G

SNACK 2

2   ounces of dry-roasted peanuts

1   cup of 2% chocolate milk

1   banana

CALORIES: 662; PROTEIN: 23 G; FAT: 34 G; CARBS: 66 G

DINNER

1½ servings of Chili

6   saltines

2   dill pickle spears

CALORIES: 587; PROTEIN: 51 G; FAT: 19 G; CARBS: 53 G

CHILI

SERVES 4

1   pound 90%-lean ground beef

½   cup water

1   package chili seasoning

1   16-ounce can diced tomatoes

1   can (15 ounces) kidney beans

1   can (8 ounces) tomato juice

In a large skillet over medium-high heat, cook the ground beef for 3 to 4 minutes, or until no longer pink. Drain the fat. Raise the heat to high and stir in the water, chili seasoning, tomatoes (with juice), beans (with liquid), and tomato juice. Heat to boiling. Reduce heat to low, cover, and cook for 20 minutes.

BREAKFAST

3 multigrain waffles with 3 tablespoons of lite syrup and 2 tablespoons of butter

2 links of turkey sausage

1 cup of orange juice

CALORIES: 798; PROTEIN: 22 G; FAT: 42 G; CARBS: 83 G

SNACK 1

1 plain bagel with 2 tablespoons of peanut butter

CALORIES: 502; PROTEIN: 20 G; FAT: 18 G; CARBS: 65 G

LUNCH

2 sandwiches, each made with 2 slices of multigrain bread, 1 tablespoon of mayonnaise, 1 tablespoon of Dijon mustard, 2 ounces of turkey lunchmeat, ½ cup of spinach, and 2 slices of tomato

1 large apple

CALORIES: 695; PROTEIN: 30 G; FAT: 27 G; CARBS: 83 G

SNACK 2

2 ounces of dry-roasted peanuts

1 cup of 1% milk

CALORIES: 463; PROTEIN: 22 G; FAT: 31 G; CARBS: 24 G

DINNER

1 serving of Hamburgers

⅓ cup of barbecue baked beans

CALORIES: 555; PROTEIN: 46 G; FAT: 19 G; CARBS: 50 G

HAMBURGERS

SERVES 4

1½ pounds 90%-lean ground beef

4 multigrain rolls

4 teaspoons ketchup

4 teaspoons mustard

8 slices dill pickle

1 large tomato, cut into 4 slices

Coat a grill rack or broiler pan with nonstick spray. Preheat the grill or broiler. Form the meat into 4 patties and place on the prepared rack or pan. Cook for 10 to 12 minutes, turning once, until a thermometer inserted in the center registers 160°F and the meat is no longer pink. Spread each roll with 1 teaspoon of the ketchup and 1 teaspoon of the mustard. Place 1 patty on each roll and garnish each with 2 slices of pickle and 1 slice of the tomato.

BREAKFAST

2 cups of Shredded Wheat and Bran with 1 cup of 1% milk

2 links of turkey sausage

¾ cup of blueberries

CALORIES: 662; PROTEIN: 33 G; FAT: 14 G; CARBS: 101 G

SNACK 1

1 cup of fruit yogurt

2 ounces of dry-roasted peanuts

CALORIES: 570; PROTEIN: 22 G; FAT: 30 G; CARBS: 53 G

LUNCH

2 sandwiches, each made with 2 slices of multigrain bread, 1 tablespoon of mayonnaise, 1 tablespoon of sweet pickle relish, and ½ can of tuna (drained)

1 medium orange

CALORIES: 729; PROTEIN: 50 G; FAT: 29 G; CARBS: 67 G

SNACK 2

2 ounces of dry-roasted peanuts

1 banana

CALORIES: 481; PROTEIN: 15 G; FAT: 29 G; CARBS: 40 G

DINNER

1 serving of Broiled Shrimp Scampi

3–5 spears (¼ pound) of boiled or steamed asparagus

1 multigrain roll with 1 tablespoon of butter

CALORIES: 475; PROTEIN: 29 G; FAT: 23 G; CARBS: 38 G

BROILED SHRIMP SCAMPI

SERVES 4

1 pound raw shrimp, peeled and deveined

¼ cup olive oil

2 teaspoons minced garlic

2 teaspoons lemon juice

¼ teaspoon salt

¼ teaspoon ground black pepper

2 tablespoons grated Parmesan cheese

Preheat the broiler. Rinse the shrimp and pat dry. In a small bowl, mix together the oil, garlic, lemon juice, salt, and pepper. Toss the shrimp in the oil mixture and place on the baking sheet. Sprinkle with the cheese. Cook for 6 to 8 minutes, or until the shrimp is opaque (watch carefully). Serve immediately.

Facts for Caffeine Addicts

Until recently, nutritionists warned that caffeinated beverages, such as cola and coffee, were diuretics. Diuretics cause you to urinate more fluid than you take in, so a Diet Coke could theoretically help you win an office pissing match. Unfortunately, for every can you drank, you'd have to drink an equal or greater amount of water to stay even and avoid a net dehydration effect.

Luckily, the latest research has shown this isn't true. If you don't drink caffeinated beverages on a regular basis, they can have a diuretic effect when you do imbibe. But if, like many people, you have a cup of joe every morning or a Pepsi every day at lunch, your body gets used to the caffeine and uses the beverage as it would any other fluid.

While a caffeine habit won't negatively affect your fluid intake, it can have an unwanted impact on your caloric intake. If you usually take your coffee without cream and sugar, you're in luck: Each cup contains only 3 to 5 calories, which is basically a negligible number. If you can't drink it black and you wish to avoid the nasty symptoms of caffeine withdrawal, you'll have to resort to stealing little packets of artificial sweeteners from restaurants. And if you're really clever, you can also spike it with some of the 1%-milk ration from your meal plan.

Cola, meanwhile, has the potential to wreak much more havoc on your T eating plan: A single can of Coke contains about 17 teaspoons of sugar. Switch to either diet soda or unsweetened iced tea.

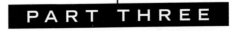

PART THREE

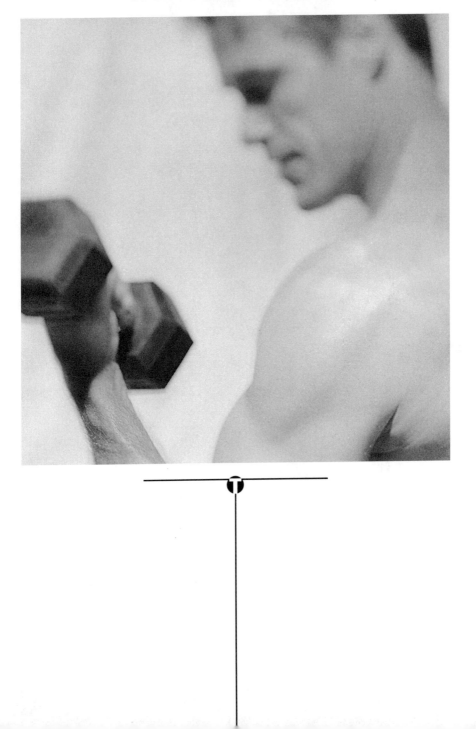

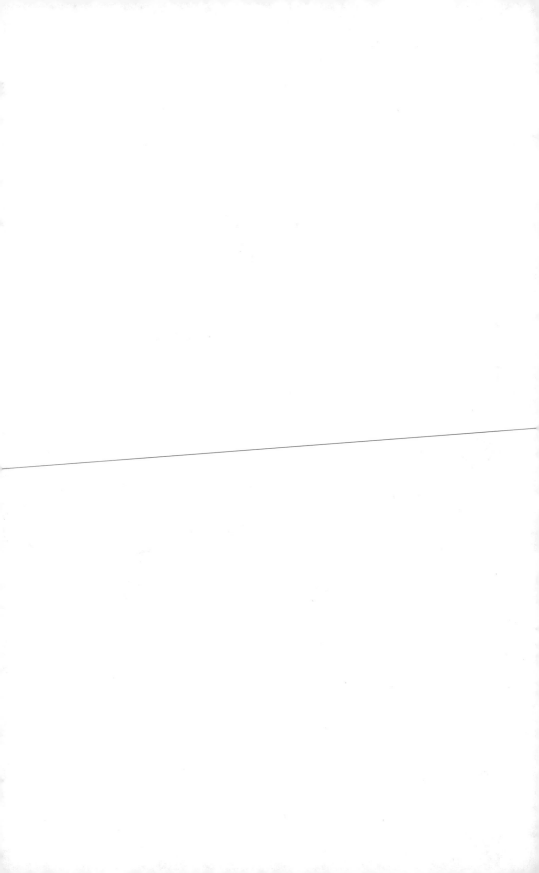

CHAPTER

12

Introduction to the Testosterone Advantage™ Workout

*A*t any given moment, on any given day, in any given gym, a buff guy is sharing the greatest wisdom he can impart: "Diet is 90 percent of the equation. You can work out from now till doomsday, but unless you get your diet in order, you aren't going to see the best results."

Learning this is sort of a rite of passage in American gyms. The day someone tells you about the 90-percent solution is the day you become a member of the club, a fellow ironworker.

Unlike a lot of gym lore, this advice has some scientific truth behind it. Let's say a guy is trying to shed fat but doesn't want to give up any of his favorite foods or otherwise change any of his eating habits. What are his chances of getting significantly leaner?

Assuming he's not a gun-toting rap star, they're about the same as his chances of adding Jennifer Lopez's name to his list of female conquests.

A review published in *Nutrition* in 2000 looked at 68 diet-and-exercise studies and came to the following conclusions.

 Exercise has little to no effect on weight loss if all you do is follow the typical guideline of 3 to 5 hours a week of moderate to vigorous activity. Studies that compared diet alone with diet coupled with minimum amounts of exercise showed that people lost about the same amount of weight either way.

👕 Exercise, however, ensures that more of the lost weight comes from fat and that more muscle is preserved. Remember, we've been careful in this book to make a clear distinction between "weight loss" and "fat loss." Pretty much everybody wants the latter. Not everybody wants the former. Especially not men.

👕 Of all types of exercise, resistance training leads to the most muscle preservation. In some studies it has even produced a simultaneous increase in muscle tissue and loss of fat, when coupled with a calorie-reduced diet.

The 90-percent argument is starting to look a little better here, isn't it?

But suppose we take another slant on it. At a recent bodybuilding conference, trainer and nutritionist Thomas Incledon, R.D., of Plantation, Florida, pulled out this real-world example: "Let's say I take two groups of Olympic weight lifters, and I give one a perfect diet with no exercise and the other a great workout with a junk-food diet. Who's going to lift more weight?"

Obviously, the guy who's training is going to perform better in this example. Diet is almost meaningless. But what if his goal consists of looking good—having the most muscle with the least fat? Here the result would probably be a push. The guy with the perfect diet and no workout is going to be thin, weak, and soft. The guy with the perfect workout and lousy diet is going to be bigger and stronger—and probably fatter.

We don't mean to confuse you beyond all imagining. We're simply trying to drive home a very important—indeed, critical—point: You probably won't like the results of the Testosterone Advantage Plan unless you're willing to expend effort on both the diet and exercise portions.

So let's assume that each element is about half of the equation. By now, of course, you know it's not quite that straightforward. As we've noted, weight training is a dynamic process. Aside from what it does to your muscles directly, it spurs changes inside your body that give rise to a multiplier effect, making you leaner faster and more dramatically. (That's the basis of the metabolic weight control we discussed in previous chapters.) But in oversimplified form, merely for the purposes of understanding why we designed the plan the way we did, you can look at it this way:

The diet controls your base weight—up, down, or sideways.

The workout distributes that weight—more muscle up in your chest, shoulders, back, and arms; less fat down in your midsection.

We've already told you everything we can about the diet. Now it's time to take a closer look at the second half of the equation.

THE T WORKOUT: HOW IT WORKS

Everyone benefits from getting stronger. Even if you (a) have no idea how much you can bench press and (b) couldn't care less, you have to admit you'd rather be able to work with more weight on basic exercises like biceps curls. Suppose you could do sets of 10 curls with 75 pounds instead of 65. Don't you think your arms would get bigger and you'd get more benefit from the same amount of time and effort in the gym?

Yet almost no one goes to the gym with the goal of just getting stronger—they go to look better. You see teenagers heaving around iron like it's their dads' charge cards, but you almost never see adults consciously trying to lift heavier weights just for the sake of lifting heavier weights, unless they're into strongman competitions. If you see an average 30-year-old guy in the gym doing bench presses with 135 pounds, chances are, you could walk into that same gym 12 months later and see that now-31-year-old guy doing bench presses with that same 135 pounds. Unfortunately, that 31-year-old guy won't look one bit better

(continued on page 160)

How Strong Can You Get, Anyway?

Our goal in this book is to help you maximize what nature gave you to work with—the operative phrase being *what nature gave you*. You can't beat yourself up over your inability to keep pace with your friend John, because John may have hardwired biological advantages over you.

Feel-good mantras about how "you can do whatever you set your mind to" are useful in certain settings. The reality, however, is that most of the factors affecting strength are inherited from Mom and Dad, right along with eye color and height. Truth be told, this applies to athleticism in general.

Here are some of the genetic factors that affect your progress in the gym.

Are You a Slow-Twitch or Fast-Twitch Kinda Guy?

You have two kinds of muscle fibers: *slow-twitch* and *fast-twitch*. Slow-twitch fibers generate small levels of force for long periods of time and thus are better suited for endurance activities. Fast-twitch fibers produce high levels of force for short bursts and are best suited for power activities. Though you should have a good balance of both, some people inherit a high percentage of one or the other—thus, at least in part, accounting for the world-class athletes who excel in given realms. (Your Olympic cross-country skiers would tend to be slow-twitch kinds of guys.) Both types of fibers respond to strength training, but generally, you get better, faster results with a higher percentage of fast-twitch fibers.

How Long Are Your Limbs?

Having trouble finding shirts whose sleeves fit? You may also have trouble keeping up with your stubby-armed lifting buddy. A guy with short arms and legs tends to be able to lift more weight in exercises like the squat and the bench press because he has better leverage, and he doesn't have to lift the weight as far. A guy with long arms and short legs has an advantage in the deadlift since he doesn't have to lift the weight as high off the floor. (For the record, this also explains why some pitchers have control problems: The longer the arm, the longer the arc; and the longer the arc, the more that can go wrong in the delivery.)

How Long Are Your Muscles?

What we said about your limbs applies here, too, but in the opposite way. If you have long muscles, you have more potential for developing size and strength than people with short muscles, and you have more muscle exerting force over a greater percentage of the limb.

The most challenging genetic configuration, therefore, is short muscles in long arms. You can tell if your muscles are short or long by counting the number of fingers you can fit between the end of your biceps and your elbow when your arm is fully flexed. If it's more than two, you have short to medium muscles. If the biceps goes to the elbow, you're a god.

Where Do Your Tendons Attach?

Even if two men closely resemble one another in every other physiological respect (percentage of muscle fibers, length of arms, length of muscles), the attachment point of their tendons to their muscles could nonetheless cause one to be substantially stronger than the other. In fact, that's one reason why competitive power-lifters typically outlift bodybuilders, who are usually much bigger muscle-wise. A tendon that attaches a bit farther up the bone from the joint provides a slight advantage because it effectively shortens the length of the limb.

How Old Are You?

You may have heard that if you're past a certain age—40 is often mentioned—you can't create new muscle. Untrue. However, if you're 40 and your lifting buddy is 20, don't expect to match his muscle-building progress vein for vein. Several studies seem to correlate the maximum rate of strength and muscle gain with the years of puberty. After you've fully come of age, you're working against your body's inherent tendency to remain at a steady state or even shed muscle mass. So the older you get, the slower you build muscle.

Once you diagnose and accept your physiology, you can develop a body-type-specific program that addresses your individual goals and capabilities. What we said earlier about genetics is true enough, but there are no limits on how much you work out, how intelligently you work out, what you eat to support your workouts, and how you live your life in general. A dedicated guy with more than his share of slow-twitch fibers will outperform a guy with an abundance of fast-twitch fibers who spends his days sprawled on the couch with a six-pack—and we're not talking about the abdominal kind.

than his 30-year-old self. He may even look worse since a body that doesn't get new stimulation will generally lose muscle mass as well as experience a slowdown in metabolism that could lead to more fat storage.

If you want to get bigger and stronger and better-looking—especially in a relatively short time period, such as the 9 weeks covered by the T plan—you need to give your muscles stimulation that's different from anything they've experienced. After a while, your muscles learn to do the same old exercises more efficiently, thus exercising a smaller amount of tissue at less intensity. For these reasons, when our co-author Michael Mejia designed the T workout program, he came up with a workout configuration that will be new to almost everyone.

Mike's second consideration in creating the T workout was time limitation. We figure 3 hours a week is the most we can ask anyone to spend lifting weights.

Finally, there was the issue of boosting testosterone. We wanted to make sure the workout that Mike created gave guys the best chance to let the big T dog do its work. So let's look at that in more detail.

THE MUSCLE/TESTOSTERONE CONNECTION

A great body is built two ways: by building muscle, and by preventing muscle from degrading. T is thought to have a number of indirect effects on muscle growth. One of these is the conversion of muscle fibers. Your body has two main types of fibers: Type I, or slow-twitch, used mostly in endurance exercise; and Type II, or fast-twitch, which are mostly used in weight lifting and have the greatest growth potential. Fast-twitch fibers, in turn, come in two types: power-oriented Type IIb fibers, used in the quickest and shortest-lasting bursts of exertion (throwing a shot put, for example), and growth-oriented Type IIa fibers, the ones that sustain you during a typical weight-lifting set.

Of all your body's fibers, Type IIa have the most potential to get bigger, and over the course of a weight-lifting program, your body converts your IIb's to IIa's, giving you more fibers that have the potential to grow larger. What makes this conversion happen? T is one of the triggers, theorize researchers Steven J. Fleck, Ph.D., chair of the department of sports medicine at Colorado College in Colorado Springs, and William J. Kraemer, Ph.D., director of the Human Performance Lab at Ball State University in Muncie, Indiana, in their book *Designing Resistance Training Programs*.

Testosterone's greatest effect, however, may be in preventing muscle degradation. In an interesting experiment, researchers at the University of Texas Medical Branch injected healthy young men with T and then, 5 days later, tested them in a fasting state. Normally, during periods of fasting or starvation, the body pulls protein from muscle tissue to survive, giving up its muscle mass to save skin and other vital organs. But with the additional testosterone in the study, the muscles didn't give up protein. The organ-saving protein must've come from somewhere, and the researchers admit they aren't sure from where—but the major finding was that testosterone kept muscle protein from degrading.

So any mook in any gym in any city in America will tell you that more T equals more muscle and more muscle equals more T. And, in a way, that mook is right. Lots of different muscle-building programs have been shown to boost testosterone. Both of the classic weight-lifting configurations—the three-sets-of-10-repetitions bodybuilding workout and the five-sets-of-5 powerlifting workout—bump up your T levels.

Yet, as is always the case when you're dealing with a magnificent system like the human body, nothing is quite that simple. For example, even the best weight workouts increase the levels of testosterone in your blood for only an hour or two after exercise. Those levels then fall and, for up to 48 hours, tend to be even lower than your initial resting T levels. No one knows for sure yet why this happens, but some researchers theorize that a decrease in testosterone after a workout is a good thing because more of the T is being taken up by muscle tissue, where it can enhance protein synthesis. As a result of this greater uptake, the blood levels go down.

What's more, most studies have shown that weight training alone does not increase your resting (basal) T levels.

That's not what you wanted to read, is it? You wanted us to tell you that walking into a gym and throwing around some iron would magically, permanently zoom your T levels to those of a bull elephant stomping around the savannah in a rutting frenzy. If only that were true, we'd all look like Steve Reeves in *Hercules Unchained*. And there'd be a serious run on condoms-by-the-gross at Sam's Club.

However, the weight-lifting component of our program isn't intended to dramatically affect your resting T rates. That's the eating plan's job.

Furthermore, the fact that your resting T levels are more or less unaffected by the overall course of a weight-training program doesn't mean testosterone isn't helping your body build muscle and burn fat. As you work out and get bigger and stronger, your body's hormone receptors become more sensitive and are able to do more with the same amount of T. Also, the more often you activate your T receptors with small bursts of testosterone, the more efficient they get at using T. So those workout-induced bursts may be important even though they subside and return to basal levels relatively quickly.

Finally, as we've already mentioned about 300 times in this book, increasing muscle also increases metabolism, or the number of calories you burn on a minute-by-minute basis. This makes muscle your number one weapon against body fat, especially the fat that accumulates around your midsection. And excess abdominal fat lowers testosterone, so essentially, weight lifting increases testosterone's effects simply by reducing fat.

BEYOND T

As important as testosterone is when you're trying to improve your body, it's not the only hormone you need to know about. Here are some others that play vital roles.

GROWTH HORMONE (GH). This is your personal liposuction machine—the biggest cucumber in the fat-burning garden. Even more than testosterone, it mobilizes your body's fat to be used as energy.

Known as a peptide hormone, GH is released in response to many different stimuli, including holding your breath. (If you think you can use this bit of trivia to help bulk up, well—and we hate to say this, but—

don't hold your breath. The quantities you can release through breath holding aren't significant enough to have any impact on body composition.) Though your levels of all hormones rise and fall over the course of the day, GH has a unique "pulsatile" action, which means it works in spurts. The biggest spurt is at night, when you sleep.

But intense exercise causes a bonus spurt. The mechanism here is thought to have something to do with lactic acid levels. Thus, it's also linked to doing multiple sets of the same exercise, which brings muscles to the point of fatigue and triggers lactic acid buildup. This is one reason why weight lifting, which doesn't burn a huge number of calories while you're actually doing it, can ultimately lead to more fat loss than the long, steady, low-intensity aerobic workouts too many of us have turned to when we were trying to get in shape.

INSULIN. Insulin is one of those good-cop/bad-cop hormones. It's the bad cop when a lifetime of overeating and underexercising have left you insulin-resistant, or unable to properly use the insulin your body generates. Insulin resistance is part of syndrome X, otherwise known as polymetabolic syndrome—a health nightmare that includes diabetes type 2, heart disease, high blood pressure, and elevated triglycerides.

Insulin is the good cop when it comes to your post-workout meal, since it speeds sugar and protein to your muscles for refueling and repair. In fact, when you're trying to build muscle, you want to make your insulin surge and move those nutrients to your muscles as quickly as possible.

Another reason to welcome this post-workout surge is that insulin seems to be an anti-catabolic hormone, meaning it prevents muscle degradation.

CORTISOL. This stress hormone is the biggest enemy you have when trying to improve your body. Cortisol promotes fat storage, particularly in your midsection. It also signals your body to use muscle protein for energy.

In other words, it's the anti-T: It shrinks your muscles and grows your gut.

A well-designed lifting program suppresses overall cortisol levels because the more your muscles shape up, the less cortisol your body produces. In a 1999 study reported in the *Canadian Journal of Applied Physiology*, resting cortisol levels decreased 17 percent over 20 weeks of weight training, while T levels remained the same. With less cortisol to interfere with its actions, T becomes more potent.

No matter how low your resting cortisol levels, however, the anti-T rises quickly each time you work out, along with other stress hormones, such as epinephrine (also known as adrenaline). After all, exercise *is* a form of stress on your body. And the whole point of working out is to force your body to respond to a new form of stress by growing bigger and stronger. So stress hormones are an important part of the muscle-building apparatus. Your body has to recognize that it's under stress before it can make the adaptations that will lead to the results you want.

But after about 60 minutes of exercise, the effects of the stress hormones overwhelm those of the anabolic, or muscle-building, hormones. Cortisol and its partners in crime bushwhack the T and GH. Your body enters a catabolic state.

Quite literally, it's breaking down. *You're* breaking down. So your goal in the weight room is to prevent this from happening. You need to maximize the stress on your muscles in an hour or less, then get the hell out and let your body recover.

One last thing:

**Aerobics, as most people know them,
actually increase cortisol production.**

MAKING A COMEBACK

Recovery requires a number of considerations, the most important of which are these:

KNOW WHEN TO SAY WHEN. We all know guys who spend more than 2 hours a day in the gym, 5 or 6 days a week. If you're an elite athlete, you have to train this hard. If you're taking steroids, you can get away with it and see a quick benefit—you'll just pay later. But if you're not training for the Olympics or injecting hormones into your buttocks, it's tremendously counterproductive.

Most trainers today believe that shorter is better and fewer workouts are better than more. In the T workout program, you'll do three workouts a week most of the time.

EAT RIGHT, AND EAT RIGHT AWAY. We covered this in part two, but it bears repeating: You need to eat some protein and carbohydrate an hour or two before a workout and then again right after training. The pre-workout protein spares the protein in your muscles, while the carbohydrate provides energy. After-workout protein and carbs stimulate insulin release, which, as we mentioned earlier in this chapter, express-delivers the nutrients to your muscles for reconstruction and reenergizing.

WORK HARD, AND REST HARDER. We give you tough workouts in the T program. But it's up to you to do what it takes to recover from them. That means maintaining consistent sleep patterns, staying away from alcohol as much as possible, drinking enough water, and limiting stress whenever you can. It also means following the T diet, which gives you the nutrients needed to build your body, and limiting strenuous activities on the days you don't train. By strenuous activity we mean heavy-duty endurance exercise such as training for a marathon. But playing some softball or basketball won't really affect your resistance-training gains in muscle mass and strength. To be safe, though, keep your aerobic activity to under 30 minutes a day and no more than three or four times a week. Beyond that, overtraining or cortisol buildup could be a problem.

Now that you're ready to challenge your muscles with new, T-enhancing, recovery-encouraging exercises, we'll get into some of the particulars of our workout program. Secure all of your preconceived notions about working out in the overhead bins, fellas. Strap on your seat belts and get ready to take off.

In the next hundred or so pages, we're going to show you how to lift some serious tonnage.

Getting Ready to Lift

Your 9-week T workout program has three phases: anatomical adaptation, hypertrophy, and strength.

ANATOMICAL ADAPTATION. For 2 weeks, you'll do circuit routines, which means you'll do one set of 15 to 20 repetitions of each exercise in the workout, then repeat once or twice. (If none of the preceding sentence made any sense at all, see "The Absolute-Beginner's Guide to Gym Terminology" on page 190. In less than 10 minutes, you can learn to speak like a genuine gym-going mook.)

The purpose of this phase is to get your muscles and connective tissues prepared for the heavier lifting to follow. You may experience some muscle growth during this stage, especially if you've lifted before but haven't done this type of high-repetition training—as we said in the previous chapter, giving your muscles a new stimulus almost always produces new muscle growth. Most likely, though, you'll just get a general feeling that your muscles are becoming tighter or more toned.

And you should get stronger in this stage. Your goal in each workout is to use more weight on each exercise, or at least do more repetitions with the same weight.

HYPERTROPHY. For 3 weeks, you'll do bodybuilding routines, performing two or three sets of 8 to 12 repetitions of each exercise. You'll do two different workouts on a rotating basis; and within workouts, you'll shift back and forth between exercises for muscle groups on opposite sides of your body. So you'll do a set of a chest exercise followed by a set of a back exercise, alternating until you've finished all the sets of each before moving on to the next exercise pair.

Your goal here is to rapidly increase muscle size and strength. Absolute beginners may not start to actually see increases in size until the second month of training, but strength increases should be noticeable by the second or third workout of this phase.

STRENGTH. Next you'll shift to 4 weeks of powerlifting workouts, doing as many as five sets of each exercise and never more than eight repetitions.

If you have some weight-training experience but have never done this type of heavy-duty lifting, you'll probably be amazed at the changes you'll see. You'll not only push and pull more weight than ever before but also probably see muscles popping out that you didn't know you had.

Be aware that this type of lifting helps you only if you employ perfect form. Bad lifting technique, at best, allows your body to use the wrong muscles to help lift the weights. That limits your gains in the targeted muscles. At worst, poor form knocks you out of commission with injuries to your most vulnerable areas: lower back, shoulders, or knees. That's why the following chapters devote so much space to words on and pictures of proper technique.

HOME VERSUS GYM

We present the Testosterone Advantage workout in such a way that you can do it at home or in the gym.

Some guys genuinely like gyms, some regard them as a necessary evil, and some would rather train in the basement, next to the cat's litter box. Here are some of the factors that go into the choice you make.

COST. For less than $1,000, you can set up a pretty cool home gym

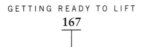

with an Olympic weight set, an adjustable weight bench, a power rack for doing heavy squats and bench presses, fixed dumbbells, and a few other workout tools. Of course, in a lot of cities, $1,000 up front buys you a multiple-year gym membership.

Advantage: Gym

MOTIVATION. Here's the biggest complaint home exercisers voice: "How do I stay pumped to pump when I'm surrounded by the same four walls?" If you find yourself asking this question, you should probably join a gym. At a good gym, the lights, room temperature, and overall surroundings are all designed to get your adrenaline flowing. Plus, you don't feel like the Lone Ranger when you're surrounded by others who share your goals. Of course, at a bad gym, you may find the lights too harsh, the room too hot or cold, and the people complete dorks. Then again, we don't know the people who share your home.

Advantage: Gym

SAFETY. Since 1996, there have been 11 reported deaths in home gyms, the most common cause being asphyxiation due to the bench press. Imagine you're trying to lift a weight, but you can't hold it up, so it comes crashing down onto your upper chest, rolls down onto your neck, and crushes your larynx. Not a pleasant thought, huh? Fortunately, this is an easy fix: Set your bench at a slight incline. This won't affect the trajectory of the lift much but will allow you to roll the bar downhill if you leave it on your chest.

Overall, the toes seem to be the body part most prone to weight-lifting injury—not actually from lifting per se but, as you might imagine, from dropping the weights . . . and that can happen in the gym as well as at home. Still . . .

Advantage: Gym

CONVENIENCE. If there's a gym in your office building, it clearly wins here. But if that's not a company perk and there's no gym on the route from your job to your home, so you have to go out of your way to get to one, the home option may work better. It's hard enough to squeeze in a good 45-minute workout without adding in drive time.

Advantage: Tie

ATMOSPHERE. The music in the gym will suck—usually some

generic rip-off of rock music that wasn't even that popular when it first came out 5 years ago. The color schemes tend to run toward purple. And as we noted earlier, if you don't like people much in general, you'll really hate the mooks and mookesses who populate the average American gym.

Advantage: Home

HYGIENE. If there's one thing worse than OPM (other people's music), it's OPS (other people's sweat). Gyms have gotten much better in recent years, either providing members with hand towels or requiring that they bring their own. Still, one gorilla wearing a stringy tank in July is all it takes to leave a bench soaked in ectoplasm. And nothing quite compares to the flora that can multiply in a communal shower stall. Your shower at home might be similarly infested with multicolored microbes, but at least they're *your* microbes.

Advantage: Home

THE WINNER: The gym, but we aren't kidding about the music. Take a Walkman.

HOW WE LABELED THE EXERCISES

We've given our exercises three separate designations: gym version, home version, and home/gym version. (You'll find the appropriate designation above the name of each exercise.) Exercises slugged "gym version," surprisingly enough, require you to have access to a gym in order to do them as shown. Exercises marked "home version" are for readers without access to a gym; if you so choose, you can follow all three phases of this program from beginning to end without ever setting foot in a health club. At the same time, obviously, the "home version" exercises also could be done in a gym—no one will scream at you if you suddenly hit the mat to reel off some pushups. In fact, even dedicated gym rats may want to mix in some of these exercises for variety. We characterize them as home exercises simply for easy identification by readers who prefer to work out in their own humble abodes.

When an exercise is described as "home/gym," it means that regardless of your workout venue—home or gym—that particular exercise is the only one available to work that muscle group at that point in the plan. Obviously, it's an exercise that the home exerciser can do with the basic equipment we outline below.

TRAINING AT HOME

Here's the equipment you'll need.

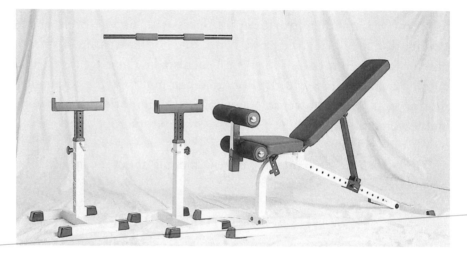

STURDY ADJUSTABLE WEIGHT BENCH WITH UPRIGHTS TO SUPPORT A BARBELL. Choose a bench that will support standard or Olympic weight sets. A lightweight bench that works only with standard weight sets won't grow with you as you get stronger; you'll need to replace it if you plan to work with heavier weights. We also recommend a bench that inclines and declines. Finally, to do all the exercises in the T workouts, you should get a bench with uprights that can be raised high enough to be used as a squat rack.

CHINUP BAR. Get a sturdy spring-loaded one that you can mount in a doorway at whatever height you need to; you can pick one up cheap at a sporting-goods store. Or build your own by using chains to hang a PVC pipe from the ceiling.

EZ-CURL BAR. This is a cambered bar that allows you to lift with your hands at 45-degree angles. A standard 1-inch bar weighs 11 pounds, while a gym version that uses Olympic weights weighs 25 pounds.

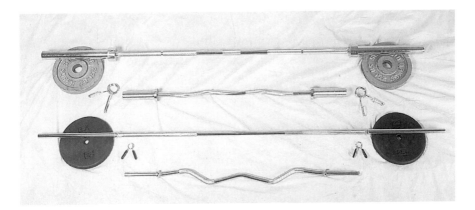

BARBELL. Most guys start with a standard 80-inch-long bar that's 1 inch in diameter and weighs 20 pounds, then move up to a 7-foot Olympic bar, which weighs 45 pounds and is the kind you most often find in commercial gyms. However, the weight plates for these bars aren't interchangeable. Standard weight plates don't fit on an Olympic bar, and vice versa.

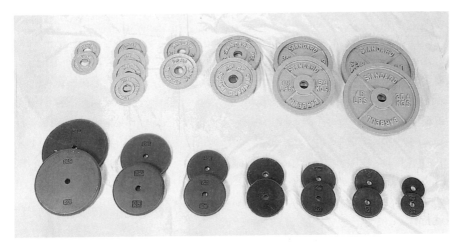

WEIGHT PLATES. Most standard sets start you off with about 90 pounds in weights, which combined with the bar will give you a total of 110 pounds to lift. You'll almost certainly have to buy extra weights to do this program. A typical Olympic set includes 280 pounds of weights in addition to the 45-pound bar.

Obviously, we think most guys are better off with an Olympic set from the get-go, but it has a few drawbacks. It takes up a lot more space, and it's very cumbersome to move a 325-pound weight set around if you need to use that space for something other than your workouts. It also may be too heavy for other members of your household to use. For example, your wife or kids may not be able to do bench presses with the 45-pound bar.

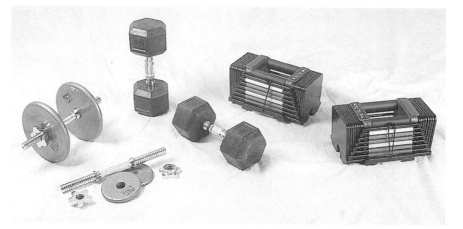

DUMBBELLS. You can get either a set of handles that lets you change weights, which makes them easy to store but clumsy and inefficient to use, or fixed dumbbells that are easy to use but take up a lot of space and get pretty pricey as you get stronger and need to use more weight. A third option is an adjustable dumbbell set like Power Blocks, which take up the same space as one set of big dumbbells but allow you to change weights quickly by moving pins back and forth. These will set you back a few hundred bucks—about the cost of an Olympic barbell set plus a pretty good collection of fixed dumbbells.

WARMING UP

You can't do the type of heavy lifting the T workout program requires without first doing a proper and thorough warmup. Cold muscles and connective tissues just can't handle it. They probably won't snap (although anything is possible when muscles are not ready for intense exercise), but they will endure damage that accumulates and can eventually lead to a serious—even debilitating—injury.

On top of that, your body simply won't perform as well if it's not properly prepared. That means less muscle for your effort.

Warmup is actually one of the few words in the gym lexicon that explains itself (unlike, for instance, *lexicon*). Your primary goal is to raise your body (core) temperature a few degrees. This allows the individual filaments in your muscles to slide back and forth easily when stretching and contracting, and it adds crucial flexibility to the tendons and ligaments that connect your muscles to your bones and your bones to each other.

Also, your knee and shoulder joints contain a substance called synovial fluid, which becomes more viscous as your temperature rises. This means your bones and connective tissues slide more easily over and around each other: Imagine well-lubricated pistons in a car engine, and you get the idea.

Just don't let the warmup become a workout in itself. Too many guys spend 20 minutes on a stairclimber, then another 5 to 10 minutes stretching. By the time they're done warming up, they're exhausted.

And more to the point, *they still haven't prepared their bodies for heavy weight lifting.*

There's no problem with doing a few minutes on a treadmill or exercise bike to help bring up your temperature. This can be your first step in warming up; however, it may not be necessary if any of the following apply.

❂ It's a warm day, and you're sweating before you get into the gym.

❂ You've walked a few blocks to get to the gym.

❂ You wear a heavy sweat suit for the start of your workout.

All these tricks should raise your core temperature enough to get you ready for strenuous exercise. Conversely, a hot shower will raise only your surface temperature. It's not a bad trick to help you wake up if you train early in the morning, but it's not an actual warmup.

(continued on page 178)

High-Test Herbs and Such

You've seen the ads. You've read the testimonials. You've looked askance at the photos of skinny "hard-gainers" and red-faced slobs who've morphed into competitive bodybuilders seemingly overnight. Like the snake-oil spiels of old, these ads are used to sell every type of nutritional supplement. Increasingly, though, the miracle-makeover claims are being applied to T-boosting supplements, the implication being that these products can have steroidlike effects.

So far, the scientific evidence behind T-elevation via supplement isn't particularly compelling or convincing. Most studies fail to show significant increases in testosterone levels—and some show scary side effects, like a link to reduced HDL levels.

We don't blame you if you're intrigued by the premise of these products. Maybe guys in your gym swear they work. Maybe you have a nutritional deficiency that the supplement corrects, allowing you to gain muscle.

On the other hand, even if rigorous scientific investigation has proven that a supplement does work, you may not respond to the product. For example, one of our co-authors participated in three creatine studies while in graduate school and, wimp that he is, never saw any im-provements in strength or muscle mass. (Not to say that creatine is considered a T-booster; we're just using it as an example of how the response to any given product differs from one guy to the next.) Scientists even have a name for unfortunates such as our intrepid scribe: nonresponders. We prefer to call them paupers since they usually end up tithing a significant portion of their take-home pay before they realize the supplement isn't doing what they'd hoped it would.

Here's what we know now—emphasis on the *now*—about the more popular T-boosting supplements. Bear in mind that the supplement industry changes quickly. By the time you read this, new studies may have come out. (If it weren't for ever-evolving research, we'd all be a bunch of carb-loading runners, feeling smug about our breakfasts of bagels and jam and wondering when the muscular guy eating sausage and eggs is going to drop dead.)

PROHORMONES. Prohormones are chemical precursors to hormones. The two you've heard the most about—androstenedione and androstenediol—are chemicals that your body naturally makes and then converts to testosterone. The idea behind prohormone supplements is that by goosing the precursors to testosterone, you'll increase the big T dog itself.

So why not just take testosterone? Because it's an illegal steroid, of course. So why aren't its precursors illegal? First, because most people had never heard of them before the summer of 1998, when a bottle of androstenedione was discovered in slugger Mark McGwire's locker during his record-breaking power surge. And second, because they don't seem to have the same effect as T.

Studies of androstenedione supplements have shown that the recommended dosages don't improve body

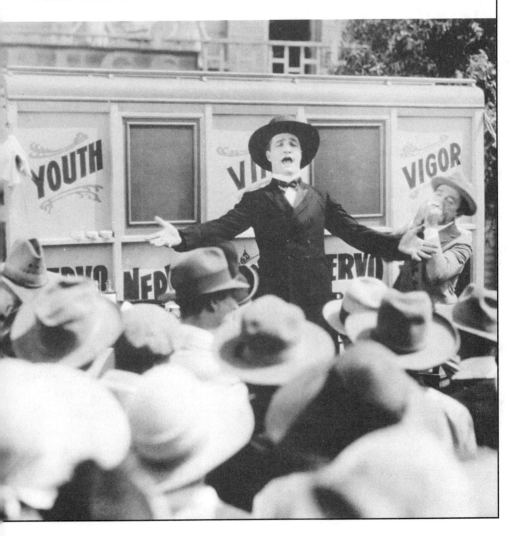

(continued)

composition (the percentage of fat versus muscle) or strength. They do, however, increase estrogen levels. And estrogen, in men, has been associated with increased risk for heart disease as well gynecomastia, better known as breast growth. (Can you imagine Big Mac with a pair of big 'uns?)

For most of us, the thought of needing to wear a "manssiere" is reason enough to avoid androstenedione. But now two other prohormones, androstenediol and norandrodiol, have attracted some buzz in gym culture. Word of mouth has it that androstenediol gives you more steroidlike effects than androstenedione, without the boost in estrogen. And norandrodiol (precursor to nortestosterone) is said to have a similar effect. This hormone is naturally produced only in animals. When taken in supplement form by humans, it's said to build muscles the same way that illegal steroids do, without such side effects as hair loss. No studies have been done yet in humans.

The bottom line is that we don't know of any solid scientific evidence showing that these claims are valid. Proponents of prohormones will tell you that if you want to see steroidlike effects, you have to take higher doses than those recommended on the labels. But legitimate researchers don't want to endanger their

study participants by having them take potentially dangerous doses. So, in other words, the doses that could show positive results will probably never be studied by mainstream researchers.

Our recommendation is that you stay away from prohormones until someone can make a sound argument for both their effectiveness and safety.

TRIBULUS. This herb comes from a plant found in Asia. Proponents claim that studies have shown tribulus to raise levels of luteinizing hormone, which would in turn raise T levels in men. However, these studies haven't appeared in peer-reviewed scientific journals, so it's impossible to assess their validity one way or the other.

Two studies that were published in legit journals failed to discover any reason to use this supplement. The first examined the effects of tribulus when consumed with androstenedione as compared with those of andro taken by itself. It found no evidence that tribulus helps to increase testosterone, reduce the estrogenic effects of androstenedione, or enhance strength compared with andro alone.

The second looked at how tribulus might affect body composition and exercise performance and found that it didn't do much for either.

One good thing you can say about tribulus is that it's been used for years in Europe and Asia, and it's probably safe, although you should use it only under the guidance of a qualified practitioner. But "safe" and "effective" aren't the same thing. Until a compelling U.S. study shows some benefits, we're going to give tribulus a pass.

ZMA. This combination of zinc (30 milligrams), magnesium (450 milligrams), and vitamin B_6 (10.5 milligrams) shows promise, according to a study published in 2000 in the *Journal of Exercise Physiology*. A group of football players at Western Washington University in Bellingham each took ZMA before bed each night during spring football—an intense, 8-week training period. Another group took a placebo. The placebo group saw their free T levels (the part your body actually uses) drop 10 percent—a reaction you'd expect during 2 months of brutal football practice. But the group taking ZMA actually increased their free testosterone by 33 per-

cent and also increased significantly in some measures of strength and power.

Now, before you grab your keys and head for the store, we have to note a pretty important conflict: One of the authors of the study is Victor Conte, who invented the supplement. That doesn't mean it wasn't a sound study or that the results necessarily were tainted. It just means that one of the guys conducting the research had a significant stake in the outcome.

The main reason we like this supplement is that there's good logic behind it. Physically active guys probably don't get enough zinc and magnesium in their diets. Both minerals are linked to T production, and both have been shown to decrease levels of the stress hormone cortisol.

One caution: Higher zinc doses may lower the body's copper content, which has led to the degeneration of heart muscle in animals. This hasn't been proven in humans, though, and the amounts of magnesium and B_6 in ZMA aren't associated with any negative side effects.

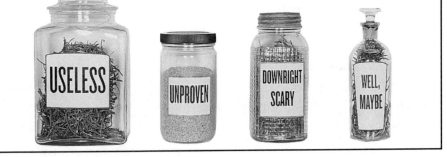

Once you've raised your core temperature, no matter how you did it, you can move on to the most crucial part of the procedure, which is getting your body ready for specific lifts. This does more than just warm up your muscles and joints. It alerts your nervous system to the type of load you're about to put on it, making your first set of exercises productive as well as painless.

Here's a foolproof warmup technique.

1. Decide how much weight you want to use in the first set of your first exercise. Let's say your routine starts with the bench press. You're a pretty good lifter, and you're going to use 185 pounds for five repetitions.

2. Do your first warmup set with about a third of that weight: 65 pounds is close enough. Do six repetitions at the lifting tempo recommended in your workout. (Your tempo will change in different Phases of the program.)

3. For your second warmup set, use half of your first-set weight: Round it off to 95 pounds. Do four repetitions at the recommended tempo.

4. Use about three-quarters of your first-set weight for two repetitions: 135 pounds will do.

5. Load the bar with 185 pounds for your first set, and rest for a minute or two.

Then you can finally take off your sweatshirt and do your first set. After such a long buildup, the actual set will be a relief, if not borderline orgasmic.

On subsequent exercises, do warmup sets when you see fit. If you switch to an exercise for a completely different muscle group—from squats to seated shoulder presses, for example—repeat the entire muscle-warmup procedure. But if you go from squats to leg presses, you need only do one set of six reps with 50 percent of the weight you intend to use.

STRETCHING

Stretching is controversial. It's almost surreal to think that a form of exercise so many people avoid is a subject of hot debate among researchers and trainers. Prescriptions are as varied as election-year tax-cut proposals, ranging from insistence that stretching should be complex and exotic to apathy about whether stretching matters much at all.

We'll say straight up that we do think it's important to stretch, and beginning on page 183, we'll show you some stretches that will help you get better results from the T program.

But we don't recommend it for the reasons you might think. So let's look at a few traditional assumptions about stretching.

- Stretching prevents injuries.
- Stretching relieves soreness and postexercise pain.
- Stretching improves sports performance.

Amazingly, each of these assumptions is backed by mostly anecdotal evidence. Research is a big coin toss. Heads, stretching works for all these purposes; tails, it doesn't.

Canadian sports-medicine specialist Ian Shrier, M.D., Ph.D., reviewed the existing studies on stretching and concluded that any type of warmup prevents injuries, regardless of whether it includes stretches. He also found no conclusive evidence that stretching relieves stiffness or soreness for more than a half hour or so, although certain types of stretches do seem to have a pain-relieving effect. This, however, could be good or bad. If a few pre-exercise stretches help you push a little past your comfort zone to achieve greater benefits from the exercise you're doing, it's good. But if they mask pain that signals the start of an injury, it's bad.

As for improving sports performance, there may be a stronger argument in favor of stretching. Mark Noble, a certified strength-and-conditioning specialist and a flexibility consultant to Duke University's perennial-powerhouse basketball team, concluded that there was a correlation between increases in flexibility and improved performance. His impetus was seeing his Blue Devils beaten by a team of European athletes whose strides seemed longer than his players', allowing them to get to the ball quicker, throw more effective screens, and get into better position for rebounds.

To put his team on an equal footing, Noble used a fairly simple series of stretches everyone knows, performed for 5 minutes twice a day. The result was improved player performance from 1987 to 2001.

STRETCHING AND STRENGTH TRAINING

Studies have shown that weight lifting, by itself, has either a positive effect or no effect on flexibility. In a 1990 study, ballet dancers actually increased their flexibility after they added weight lifting to their training program.

In other words, as we pointed out in chapter 3, the idea that weight lifting will make you "muscle-bound," and thus chronically stiff and needing additional flexibility exercise, is flat-out wrong.

Now, it *is* true that you can succeed at training yourself into inflexibility by following a poorly designed exercise program that emphasizes one muscle group without compensating with equal exercise for the opposite muscles. So you may see chronic bench pressers with pectorals so tight that their shoulders round forward.

That won't happen to you with the T program; it carefully balances exercises for complementary muscle groups.

So why are we telling you to stretch? Not because you'll prevent injuries—a thorough warmup and proper lifting form do that. Not because we think lifting makes you inflexible or unbalanced—that won't happen in a well-designed program. We think stretching, at the right time and in the right way, helps you use more muscle in any given exercise. Using more muscle means building more muscle. Building muscle increases metabolism, which decreases fat, which indirectly increases testosterone.

If that sounds like a leap, here's just one scenario in which stretching combined with strength training helps you build more muscle than strength training alone does: Most guys are pretty inflexible in the muscles around their hip joints, particularly the hip flexors (on the fronts of their pelvises) and piriformis (on the outsides of their gluteals). Tightness in these muscles limits your range of motion on the squat. And the deeper you go on the squat, the harder you work your gluteal muscles, according to our co-author Dr. Volek. Thus, more flexibility equals a better workout for the biggest muscles on your body. And working the biggest muscles not only provides the biggest post-workout T boost but also gives you the biggest metabolic benefit: more calories burned at rest.

Not bad for a few minutes of daily stretching.

Here are the specifics of our stretching program.

WHEN TO STRETCH

Because of time limitations, many guys stretch either after their weight workouts or at another time entirely. For example, they may do cardiovascular exercise on separate days from their weight workouts and stretch right after that, when their muscles are warm. (You don't have to wait for your muscles to be warm to stretch. You just can't stretch them as aggressively when they're cold.)

Many trainers have their athletes stretch before lifting, following a short, low-intensity aerobic warmup. For example, Australian strength coach Ian King has his athletes stretch aggressively before weight workouts. Before a 40-minute workout, they stretch for 20 minutes.

The best time for you to stretch is pretty much up to you. We're not going to make a specific recommendation. You may find you get the best results by stretching before a weight workout, when your muscles are fresh and your mind is focused. Or you may do better when you stretch on separate days and devote more time to it, without rushing through the stretches to get to the weights.

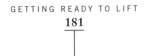

Our only firm recommendation is to find some way to work flexibility into your routine.

HOW LONG TO HOLD EACH STRETCH

Once again, we have to be equivocal here. Shrier's research found that a variety of different stretch durations produced similar results. So how much time you spend on any stretch is really a decision you make about how much attention that muscle group needs.

In general, we'd vote for a single 10- to 15-second stretch for upper-body muscles, and two or three 15- to 30-second stretches for your bigger, tighter lower-body muscles.

Yet another option, which we learned from King, is to give more attention to one side of your body than to the other. Most of us are tighter on the side we use more—our right arms and legs, if we're right-handed. So, if there's a big difference in your flexibility from one side to the other, you can do two stretches for your tight side for each one you do on your more flexible side.

THE STRETCHES

Try the following stretching sequence, holding the upper-body stretches for 10 to 15 seconds (or 10 to 15 seconds on each side, if you need to stretch both sides) and the lower-body stretches for 15 to 30 seconds (or 15 to 30 on each side). Repeat the lower-body stretches if you feel that you need to, or just repeat them on one side, if one leg is less flexible than the other.

All the one-sided stretches are described as starting with the right arm or leg. That's because most people are right-handed, and as we said above, most tend to be tighter on their dominant sides. But if you're a left-hander or the rare right-hander who's tighter on his left side, start one-sided stretches with your left arm or leg instead of your right.

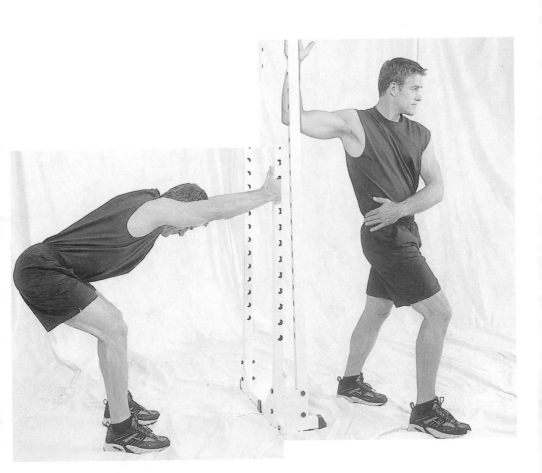

UPPER BACK
Find a sturdy bar or horizontal surface that's about chest-high. Stand 3
feet away from it, bend at the waist,
lean forward, and grip the bar.
Lower your head and chest until you
feel a good stretch in your lats.

CHEST
Stand a few feet from a wall and lean
your right forearm on it, keeping
your upper arm parallel with the
floor. Turn your torso away from
your arm just until you feel a slight
stretching in your chest. Hold for 10
to 15 seconds, then repeat with your
left arm. You should feel the stretch
across your pectoral muscles and the
fronts of your shoulders.

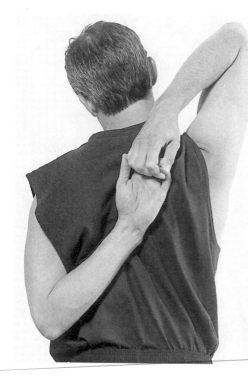

NECK AND UPPER TRAPEZIUS

Stand with feet shoulder-width apart and your knees relaxed. Keep your navel pulled in toward your spine. Reach behind your back with your right hand, keeping your forearm nearly perpendicular to the floor. Reach around your back with your left hand and grasp your right hand, gently pulling it to your left. As you do so, gently tilt your head toward your left shoulder. Feel the stretch on the right side of your neck and upper traps. Repeat on your left side.

REAR SHOULDER

Stand and reach across your chest with your right arm. Hook your left forearm behind your right elbow, and gently push your right arm across your body. Feel the stretch behind your right shoulder, then repeat on your left side.

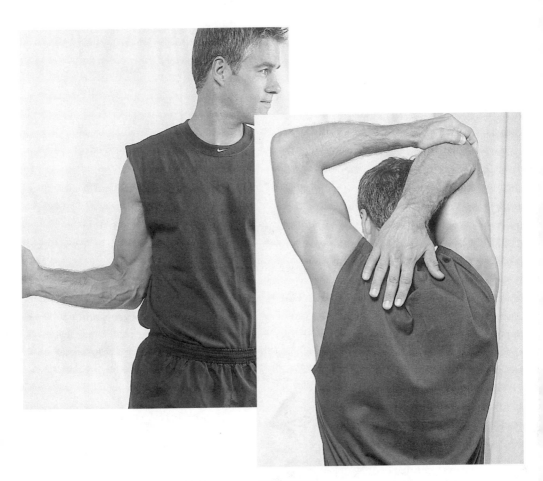

INTERNAL ROTATOR CUFF

Stand in a doorway and place your right palm and inner forearm on the right side of it, your elbow bent at a 90-degree angle. Lean forward until you feel a gentle stretch inside your right shoulder. Repeat on your left side.

TRICEPS

Stand and reach behind your head with your right hand, laying your palm flat on your upper back. Reach over your head with your left hand and place your left palm on your right elbow. Gently push the elbow down and back until you feel a stretch in your triceps. Repeat on your left side.

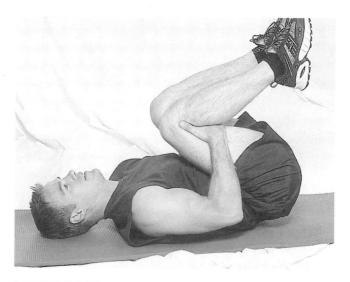

LOWER BACK

Lie on your back on a mat, bend your knees, and grab
your rear thighs just behind your knees. Pull your knees
to your chest. Shift your weight up toward your shoulders as your hips come off the floor. Feel the stretch in
your lower back.

GLUTEUS AND HIP

Lie on the mat with
your left knee bent
and your left foot on
the floor. Cross your
right leg over your
left, resting your right
ankle against your
left knee. Reach
under your left thigh
and pull your leg to-
ward your chest. Re-
peat on your right
side.

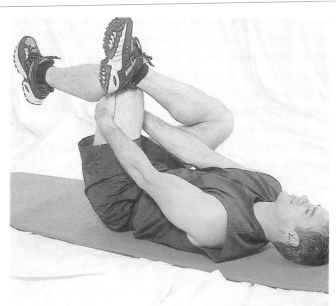

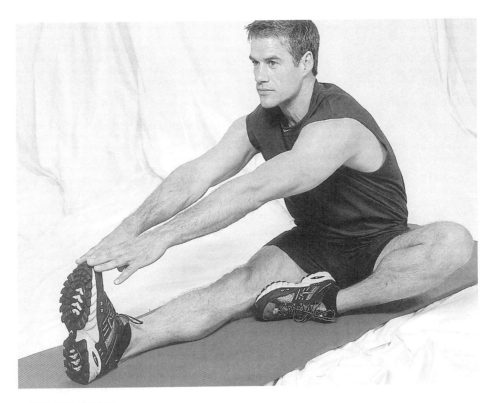

HAMSTRINGS

Sit on the mat and extend your right leg out in front of you, toes pointing up. Bend your left leg so the sole of your left foot rests against the inside of your right thigh. Keeping your back as flat as possible, lean forward and reach both hands toward your toes until you feel a gentle stretch in your right hamstrings. Repeat on your left side.

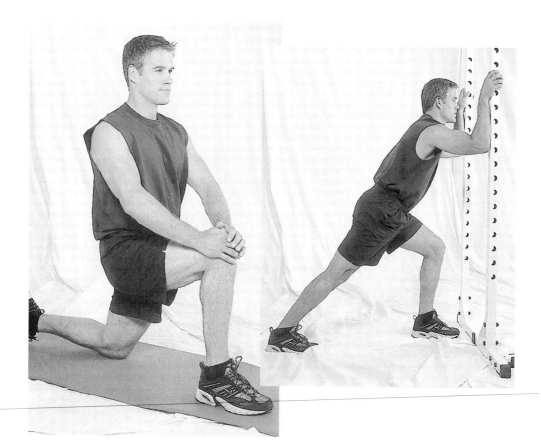

QUADRICEPS AND HIP FLEXORS

Kneel down on your left knee with your right foot about 2 feet in front of you. Tilt your pelvis forward by tucking your glutes under your torso and pulling your belly button toward your spine. Holding this pelvic position, place both hands on your right knee and shift your body weight forward until you feel a stretch in your left quad and hip flexor. Repeat on your right side.

CALF

Stand facing a wall and rest your forearms on it. Move your right foot 3 to 4 feet back. Bend your left leg and keep your right leg straight. Keeping your right heel on the floor, lean even closer to the wall until you feel a good stretch in your right calf muscle and Achilles tendon. Repeat on your left side.

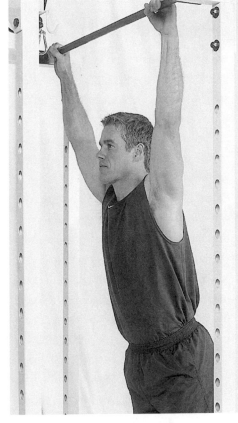

ABDOMINALS

Grab a chinup bar or the top of a doorjamb with an overhand grip. (Your feet should touch the floor, so if you use a chinup bar, you may need to stand on a bench or step). Lean forward so your weight is on the balls of your feet. Feel a stretch through the front of your body, from your forearms through the front of your shoulders to your chest, abdominals, and front hips.

SIDE TORSO

Using the same setup as for the abdominal stretch, turn to your left and grab the chinup bar or doorjamb with your palms facing one another. Lean in and rotate your body counterclockwise (to your left) until you feel a gentle stretch along the right side of your torso, down through your right hip. Repeat on your left side.

All of this should leave you feeling nice and limber—and ready to lift some serious lumber.

The Absolute-Beginner's Guide to Gym Terminology

Even those of us who've been hitting the gym for years have not forgotten that mortifying moment back in our early days of lifting—before we'd learned to talk the talk—when some mook grunted, "Gimme a spot," and we had no idea whether we were supposed to offer him a seat, wipe his brow, hand over our wallets, or perform a sexual favor. (The correct answer, as you'll soon learn, is none of the above.)

Similarly, we know there was a learning curve to figuring out which muscles were which, and which exercises worked them. We remember a particularly sad moment when a nimrod convinced us that the bench press works the lats, not the chest.

The following quick reference guide includes enough mook-speak to save you from similar embarrassment. If even the definitions use words that throw you, simply look elsewhere in this glossary, and you'll likely find them defined in their own right.

The Lingo

SPOT: Assistance on a lift, typically a bench press. A spotter stands behind a lifter and touches the bar only when the lifter clearly can't finish the lift on his own. In a well-equipped gym, the bench-press station has a platform for the spotter to stand on. A second exercise for which a spotter comes in handy is the pullup. Though it's the best exercise for overall back strength and muscular development, most guys in the gym can't do a single one. The spotter literally gives you a leg up: He stands behind you and pushes gently on your feet or ankles till you build the strength to do several.

REPETITION (REP): A single performance of an exercise. When you finally manage to get your chin up over that bar to complete a pullup, ask your spotter to congratulate you. You've done one rep.

ONE-REP MAX (1RM): The most weight you can lift once with good form. Oddly, though most guys can tell you their 1RMs for the bench press (the familiar exercise wherein you lie down and push the weight up and away from your chest), few seem to know them for any other exercise.

SET: A series of repetitions. Usually, sets are shown as a range of repetitions; for instance, 8 to 12. That means you should choose a weight that will allow you to do at least 8 reps, but no more than 12. There's a lot of trial and error involved in figuring this out.

SUPERSET: A combination of sets of multiple exercises. The most common type of superset pairs exercises for muscle groups that perform opposite functions. For example, you might do a set of bench presses followed by a set of rows (pulling exercises for your back). Another type of superset, called a *compound set*, involves two sets of exercises for the same muscle group. So you might do a set of bench presses followed by a set of dumbbell flies. A superset involving three consecutive exercises is sometimes called a *triset*. If a superset includes more than three exercises, it's usually called a *giant set*.

while leaning back on an incline bench or when you use a narrow grip on a bar.

BRACHIALIS (*NICKNAME:* NONE, REALLY—AS MUSCLES GO, IT'S NOT THE BIG MAN ON CAMPUS). This muscle lies between the upper-arm bone and the biceps, with which it shares elbow-bending duties. It works in combination with a forearm muscle called the *brachioradialis*, which is the muscle that's on top of your forearm when your palm faces the floor. The best exercises for developing the brachialis are curls using a neutral, or hammer, grip (in which your palms face your torso).

(continued)

The Muscles

BICEPS (*NICKNAMES:* BI'S AND, WHEN REFERRING TO THE ENTIRE ARM, GUNS).

The uppermost upper-arm muscle, it's one of two muscles that are responsible for bending your arm at the elbow. It has two parts: The innermost section, also called the *short head*, gets the most work when you're doing a barbell biceps curl with a medium or wide grip. The outer section, or *long head*, works more when you do a curl

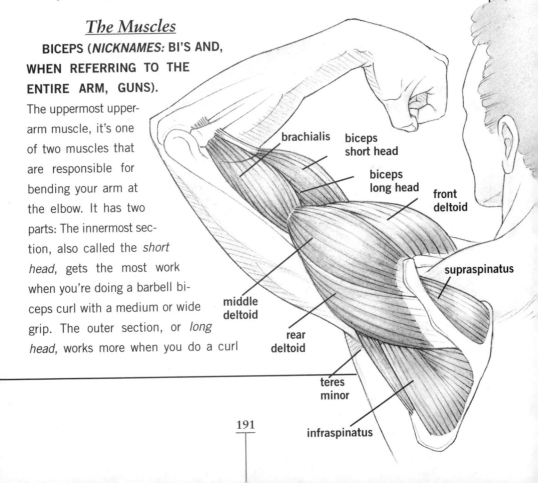

brachialis

biceps short head

biceps long head

front deltoid

supraspinatus

middle deltoid

rear deltoid

teres minor

infraspinatus

The Absolute-Beginner's Guide to Gym Terminology (cont.)

TRICEPS (*NICKNAMES:* TRI'S AND, WHEN WELL-DEVELOPED AND VISIBLE AS AN INVERTED *U* JUST BENEATH YOUR DELTOID, HORSESHOE). This rear upper-arm muscle has three parts: the *lateral head* (on the outside), the *long head* (on the inside), and the *medial head* (beneath the long head). Its job is to straighten your arm out of a bent position.

ROTATOR CUFF (*NICKNAME:* ROTATOR). The rotator cuff includes four small shoulder muscles. The *subscapularis* is involved in internal rotation (as in throwing a baseball or football); the *infraspinatus* and *teres minor* are responsible for external rotation (as in cocking your arm back before throwing); and the *supraspinatus* helps the middle deltoid muscle raise your arm to the side (as in a lateral raise). In weight lifting, the external rotators are most easily injured, so in this program you'll do specific exercises to preemptively strengthen them.

DELTOIDS (*NICKNAMES:* DELTS, CAPS, COCONUTS, AND—WHEN EXTREMELY WELL-DEVELOPED—CANNONBALLS). These are your shoulder muscles, and they consist of muscle fibers that assist in three separate actions: Your *front deltoids* lift objects when your arms are in front of your body, as in a front dumbbell raise or a chest press; your *middle deltoids* lift your arms up to your sides, as in a lateral raise; and—we bet you can guess this next term—your *rear deltoids* pull your arms back when they're perpendicular to your torso, as in a reverse fly. Both your front and middle deltoids work when you're doing an overhead shoulder press.

TRAPEZIUS (*NICKNAME:* TRAPS). A diamond-shaped muscle that runs from your middle back to the tips of your shoulder blades and up to your neck. The top of the muscle shrugs your shoulders up to your ears, the middle of the muscle pulls your shoulder blades together in back, and the lower part of the muscle pulls your shoulder blades down. Usually, the only part of this muscle that people train specifically is the upper traps, during shrugs. However, the lower part is also worked during pullups and lat pulldowns, and the middle part is worked on those two exercises and also during rows and deadlifts, even though folks don't usually think of using these exercises for this purpose. Shoulder presses also give the trapezius considerable work.

**LATISSIMUS DORSI (*NICKNAME:*

LATS). Located on the sides of your mid- and upper back. These fan-shaped muscles pull your arms down from overhead, as in a lat pulldown, or pull your body up, as in a pullup or an activity like rock climbing. They work with your biceps on many exercises.

SPINAL ERECTORS (*NICKNAME: NONE*). The *erector spinae* are the muscles that start in your lower back and snake up alongside your spine. Their job is to straighten your back when you're bent forward at the waist.

GLUTEALS (*NICKNAMES:* BUTT, GLUTES, BUNS). These are your buttock muscles: the *gluteus maximus*, which you admire on fitness babes like Kiana Tom; the *gluteus medius*, on the outside of your hip; and the *gluteus minimus*, beneath the medius. The pair of maximi (one on each cheek) straighten your hips when you're bent forward at the waist, as in a deadlift (for which they work closely with the hamstrings and spinal erectors) or squat. A single one can extend a leg backward, as in one of those butt-blaster moves that, at most gyms, only women do. The medius and minimus lift your leg straight out to the side.

(continued)

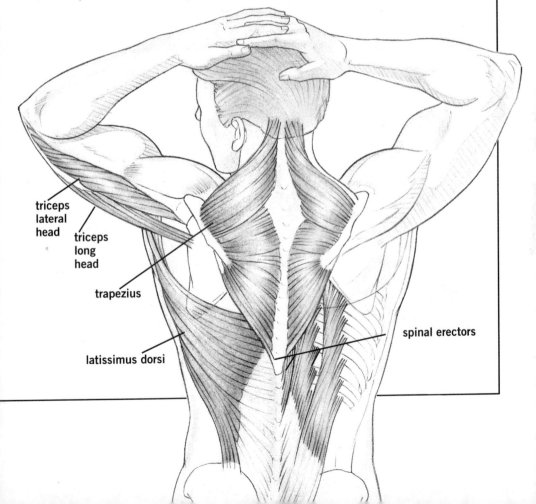

triceps lateral head

triceps long head

trapezius

latissimus dorsi

spinal erectors

PECTORALS (*NICKNAME:* PECS). The *pectoralis major* is your main chest muscle, working with your triceps and front deltoids to push a heavy object off your chest (as in a bench press—or when your girlfriend's fat damn cat jumps on you while you're lying on the sofa). The pecs also work alone to pull your arms from your sides to your midline (as in a fly). Your *pectoralis minor*, which lies beneath the pecs major and assists in its actions, pulls your shoulder blades apart, as when you fully extend your arms out in front of your chest.

ABDOMINALS (*NICKNAMES:* ABS, SIX-PACK). You have four distinct muscles here: the *rectus abdominis*, the strip that becomes a six-pack in the best-developed physiques; the *external obliques*, or the muscles on the sides of your waist; the *internal obliques*, which lie beneath the external obliques; and the *transverse abdominis*, a thin strip of muscle that, thankfully, holds your internal organs in place. Your rectus abdominis pulls your rib cage toward your pelvis, as in a crunch. Your external and internal obliques help you bend to the sides and twist at the waist. Your transverse abdominis holds everything up and in, keeping your abdomen from bulging out; you work it when you suck in your gut.

HIP FLEXORS (*NICKNAME:* NONE, AS FAR AS WE KNOW). These are the tiny strips of muscle on the front of your pelvis, consisting of the *psoas major*, *psoas minor*, and *iliacus*. They lift up your thigh in

pectoralis major

pectoralis minor

external obliques

internal obliques

psoas minor

psoas major

iliacus

transverse abdominus

rectus abdominus

front of your body, as in a leg raise. (In sports, they're involved in kicking.) The *rectus femoris*, described below under "Quadriceps," is also a hip-flexor muscle.

QUADRICEPS (*NICKNAME: QUADS*). As its name implies, this grouping of large muscles on the front of your thigh includes four parts: the *vastus lateralis* (outside front thigh), *vastus medialis* (inside front thigh), *vastus intermedius* (beneath these first two), and *rectus femoris* (top of front thigh). The first three work to straighten your knee out of a bent position, as in a squat, leg press, lunge, or leg extension. The last muscle does that and also helps lift your upper leg up in front of your body.

HAMSTRINGS (*NICKNAME: HAMS, HAMMIES*). The muscles on the back of your upper leg, including, on the outer half of your rear thigh, the *biceps femoris,* and, on the inner half of your rear thigh, the *semitendinosus* and *semimembranosus*. They have two roles: They bend your knee out of a straight position (as in a leg curl), and they straighten your hips out of a bent position (as in a deadlift). To help correct an imbalance in these muscles, turn your foot in or out during a leg curl to give more emphasis to one side or the other. Turning your foot outward emphasizes the femoris; turning it in adds work for the semitendinosus and semimembranosus.

CALVES (*NICKNAME:* GASTROCS). You have two main calf muscles: the *gastrocnemius*, the diamond-shaped outer part of the muscle, which works when you stand up on your toes with your legs straight; and the *soleus*, a thick, flat strip of muscle that lies beneath it and is responsible for lifting your heels when your knees are bent.

rectus femoris

gluteus medius

gluteus maximus

semi-membranosus

semi-tendinosus

vastus medialis

biceps femoris

vastus lateralis

vatsus intermedius

gastrocnemius

soleus

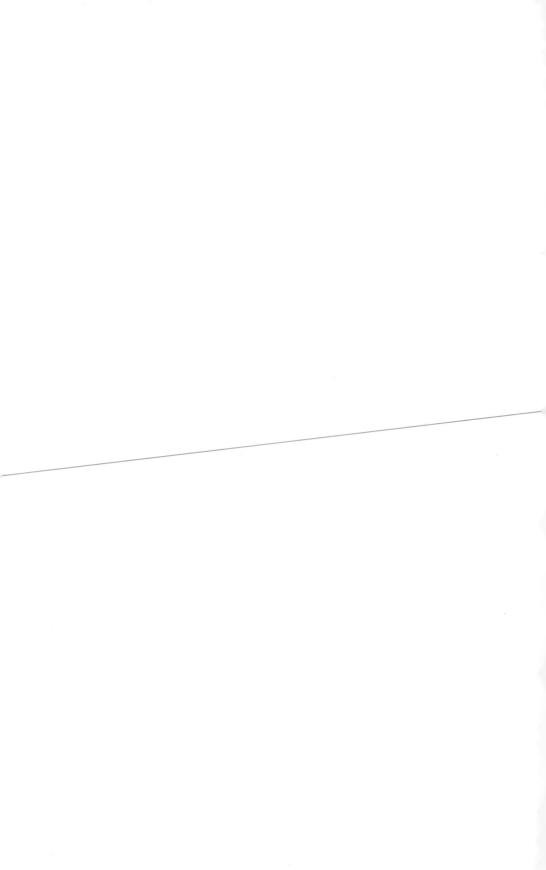

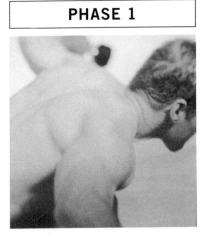

THE
TESTOSTERONE
ADVANTAGE™ WORKOUT

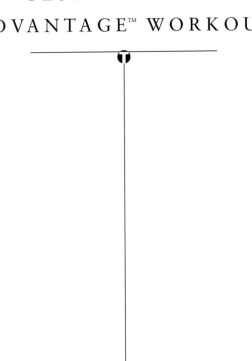

The
Testosterone Advantage™ Workout:
Phase 1

*T*hank you for entrusting us with your muscles. We hope you're raring to go. Now throw on some sweats and let's get started.

In the first 2 weeks of the T workout program, your goal is to get your body ready to build muscle. Why not go straight into the best muscle-building workouts? Because your body may not be ready. Your joints and connective tissues need prep time before they can lift heavy loads through a full range of motion. And your muscles and nerves probably aren't in sync yet, especially if you're new to weight lifting or coming back from a layoff. It takes a few weeks to learn these exercises—to coordinate muscles and nerves in an efficient way—before you can use heavier loads.

That said, these aren't weenified workouts. You'll have to work hard here. You'll sweat. You'll lose body fat, if that's your goal. Most of all, you'll get yourself good and ready for the heavier loads in the next two phases.

PHASE-1 GOAL: Anatomical adaptation

DURATION: 2 weeks

FREQUENCY: Two or three workouts per week

EXERCISES: 12

TECHNIQUE: Circuit. Complete one set of each exercise in the workout before repeating the entire circuit of exercises.

NUMBER OF CIRCUITS: Two or three per workout (two recommended in Week 1, two or three in Week 2)

WARMUP: After a brief general warmup to raise your core temperature (5 to 10 minutes at an easy pace on a treadmill, for example), use your first circuit as a more specific warmup. Use two-thirds to three-quarters of the weight you'll use on the second and third circuits. That is, if you'll use 100 pounds on the leg press, do your first circuit with 70 pounds.

REST: 1 minute between sets, 2 to 3 minutes between circuits

REPETITIONS: 15 to 20 per set. As soon as you hit 20 repetitions with a weight, increase the weight in the next workout.

TEMPO: Each set should take a little more than a minute. If you take 4 seconds to complete each repetition, a 15-rep set would take 1 minute and a 20-rep set would take 80 seconds. To get used to 4-second reps, count 2 seconds each time you lower a weight, pause for 1 second, then use the 4th second to lift the weight. If you're not familiar with the gym, it may sound backward to go slower on the lowering than on the lifting. You do this to avoid a "bounce" at the bottom of the rep. By lifting in this way, you reduce the momentum of the exercise, starting from a dead stop each time and forcing your muscles to do all the work. It's also safer since the weights are under control at all times.

THE T WORKOUT LOG

Photocopy the following pages and take them to the gym with you. Record how much weight you use and how many repetitions you perform for each exercise, for each of the three circuits you do in a workout.

Your goal is to see progress from one workout to the next: either more weight used on each exercise or more repetitions at the weight previously used. But because your muscles may be able to use more weight than your connective tissues can handle at first, limit increases to 10 percent from one workout to the next.

Phase-1 Workout

	WEEK 1			
	WORKOUT 1		WORKOUT 2	
1 **Leg press (or split squat)**	WEIGHT	REPS	WEIGHT	REPS
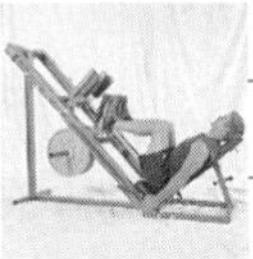 Circuit 1				
Circuit 2				
Circuit 3				
2 **Machine chest press (or pushup)**	WEIGHT	REPS	WEIGHT	REPS
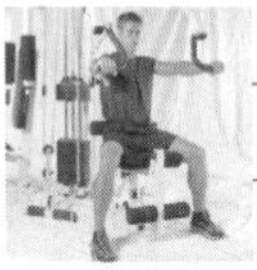 Circuit 1				
Circuit 2				
Circuit 3				
3 **Leg curl (or dumbbell leg curl)**	WEIGHT	REPS	WEIGHT	REPS
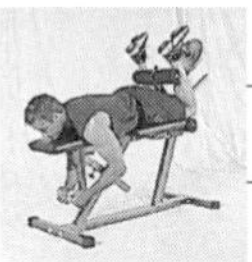 Circuit 1				
Circuit 2				
Circuit 3				
4 **Underhand-grip lat pulldown (or one-arm dumbbell row)**	WEIGHT	REPS	WEIGHT	REPS
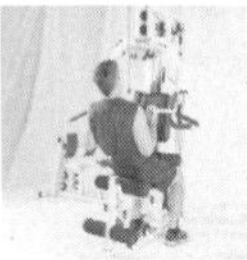 Circuit 1				
Circuit 2				
Circuit 3				
5 **Leg extension (or dumbbell leg extension)**	WEIGHT	REPS	WEIGHT	REPS
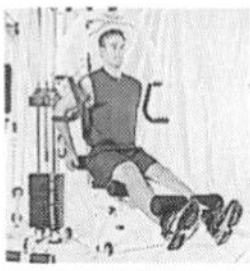 Circuit 1				
Circuit 2				
Circuit 3				
6 **Lateral raise**	WEIGHT	REPS	WEIGHT	REPS
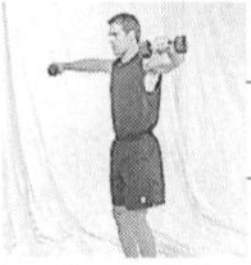 Circuit 1				
Circuit 2				
Circuit 3				

	WEEK 2						
WORKOUT 3		**WORKOUT 4**		**WORKOUT 5**		**WORKOUT 6**	
EIGHT	REPS	WEIGHT	REPS	WEIGHT	REPS	WEIGHT	REPS
EIGHT	REPS	WEIGHT	REPS	WEIGHT	REPS	WEIGHT	REPS
EIGHT	REPS	WEIGHT	REPS	WEIGHT	REPS	WEIGHT	REPS
EIGHT	REPS	WEIGHT	REPS	WEIGHT	REPS	WEIGHT	REPS
EIGHT	REPS	WEIGHT	REPS	WEIGHT	REPS	WEIGHT	REPS
EIGHT	REPS	WEIGHT	REPS	WEIGHT	REPS	WEIGHT	REPS

(continued)

Phase-1 Workout
(cont.)

	WEEK 1			
	WORKOUT 1		WORKOUT 2	
7 Standing calf raise	WEIGHT	REPS	WEIGHT	REPS
Circuit 1				
Circuit 2				
Circuit 3				
8 Machine row (or reverse fly)	WEIGHT	REPS	WEIGHT	REPS
Circuit 1				
Circuit 2				
Circuit 3				
9 Crunch	WEIGHT	REPS	WEIGHT	REPS
Circuit 1				
Circuit 2				
Circuit 3				
10 Seated dumbell biceps curl	WEIGHT	REPS	WEIGHT	REPS
Circuit 1				
Circuit 2				
Circuit 3				
11 Back extension (or Superman)	WEIGHT	REPS	WEIGHT	REPS
Circuit 1				
Circuit 2				
Circuit 3				
12 Triceps pushdown (or lying dumbbell triceps extension)	WEIGHT	REPS	WEIGHT	REPS
Circuit 1				
Circuit 2				
Circuit 3				

			WEEK 2				
WORKOUT 3		**WORKOUT 4**		**WORKOUT 5**		**WORKOUT 6**	
IGHT	REPS	WEIGHT	REPS	WEIGHT	REPS	WEIGHT	REPS
IGHT	REPS	WEIGHT	REPS	WEIGHT	REPS	WEIGHT	REPS
EIGHT	REPS	WEIGHT	REPS	WEIGHT	REPS	WEIGHT	REPS
IGHT	REPS	WEIGHT	REPS	WEIGHT	REPS	WEIGHT	REPS
IGHT	REPS	WEIGHT	REPS	WEIGHT	REPS	WEIGHT	REPS
IGHT	REPS	WEIGHT	REPS	WEIGHT	REPS	WEIGHT	REPS

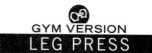

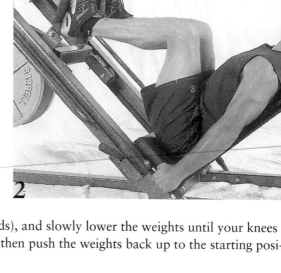

START

Position yourself in the leg press machine so your back is against the pad and your feet are about shoulder-width apart on the platform.

FINISH

Unlock the platform (usually by turning the release mechanisms outward with your hands), and slowly lower the weights until your knees are bent 90 degrees. Pause, then push the weights back up to the starting position.

DO IT RIGHT

🖜 About the only way to screw up a leg press is to lower the weights too far. If your lower back starts to come up off the pad, you know you've gone too far.

🖜 Because most of us are naturally strong in our lower bodies, it's tempting to pile on the plates. You have to exercise caution. It's okay to fudge a bit on the 10-percent rule and increase the weight by 15 percent or so from one workout to the next. But avoid the temptation to double it.

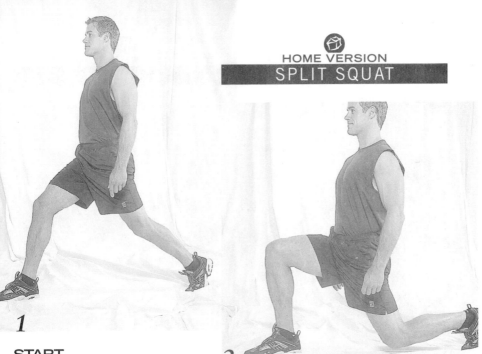

1

2

START

Stand with your feet hip-width apart, then take a long stride so your front foot is 3 to 4 feet in front of your back foot. Your toes should point forward. Keep your torso upright.

FINISH

Lower your body until your front knee is bent 90 degrees. Your front lower leg should be perpendicular to the floor, your front thigh parallel to the floor. Your rear knee should almost touch the floor, while your torso stays upright. Return to the starting position. Finish all your repetitions, then reverse legs and repeat. That's one set.

DO IT RIGHT

☉ You don't want your front knee to go past your toes as you do the exercise. Avoid this by starting with your front foot far enough forward.

☉ When you can do 20 repetitions with each leg, add weights. The best option is to hold a barbell across the back of your shoulders, but you can also hold dumbbells in your hands, at arm's length or up on your shoulders. Start light (if you're working with a barbell, use just the bar at first), then slowly increase the weight, following the 10-percent rule.

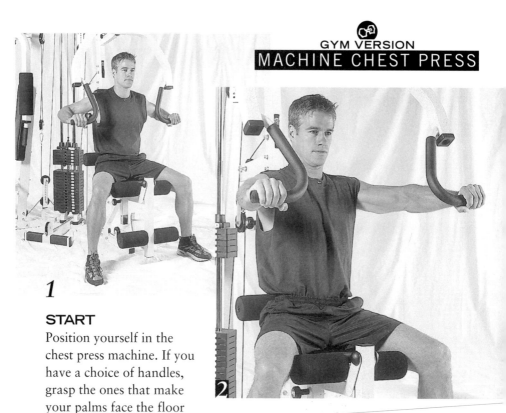

1

START
Position yourself in the chest press machine. If you have a choice of handles, grasp the ones that make your palms face the floor (not each other). This grip will ensure more chest involvement.

2

FINISH
Push the handles out until your arms are fully extended, then slowly return to the starting position.

DO IT RIGHT
⊕ There's almost no way to do this exercise wrong, but some guys try to get macho and push too much weight. If you have to arch your back, you're lifting too much.

⊕ One of the best uses of the machine chest press is in developing tempo. Try counting 1-2-3 as you lower the weight.

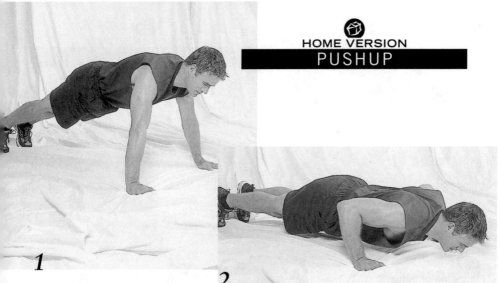

1

2

START

Balance your body on your palms and toes. Your hands should be shoulder-width apart, your feet hip-width apart. Your body should be as straight as possible from head to heels.

FINISH

Slowly lower yourself until your chest is an inch or two from the floor, then push back up to the starting position.

DO IT RIGHT

🔱 This ain't boot camp or gym class. Nobody's punishing you, and the object isn't to see how many you can do. You're trying to build muscles in your chest, triceps, and shoulders. That means slow repetitions, keeping constant tension on your muscles.

🔱 When you can do three sets of 20 pushups and make each of those sets last 80 seconds—in other words, 4 seconds per pushup—you need to make the exercise harder. Try the following variations, in this order:

Three-point pushup. Put one foot on top of the other, toes of top foot on heel of bottom foot. Switch feet from top to bottom with each set.

Decline pushup. Rest your feet on a bench, chair, couch, or slow-moving pet. This shifts the emphasis a bit to your shoulders and the top of your chest. But most important, it makes you work harder against gravity.

Decline three-point pushup. Put one foot on top of the other and both on top of a bench. If this is easy even though you haven't yet finished this 2-week phase 1, go ahead and advance to the barbell bench press described in the next phase, on page 233.

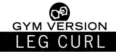

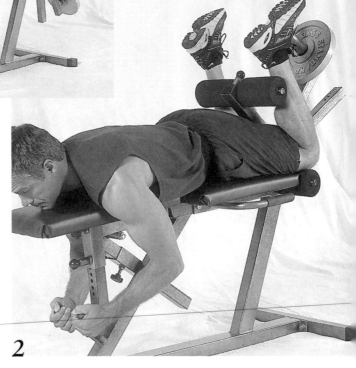

START

Lie in the leg curl machine with the leg pads against your lower legs, above your heels and below your calf muscles.

FINISH

Without raising your body off the horizontal pad, bend your legs at the knees and lift the weight as high as you can. Pause, then slowly return to the starting position.

DO IT RIGHT

🔱 You can tell you're descending into Mookville and trying to lift too much weight if you feel the exercise in your lower back. The problem is that your body doesn't want to isolate your hamstring muscles (on the backs of your thighs), so it tries to use your gluteals and lower back to help with the movement. The solution is to keep your pelvis and the fronts of your thighs in contact with the horizontal pad throughout the movement. If you have to, use lighter weight until your body gets used to the movement.

🔱 Another sign you're trying to lift too much is if your head comes up on each repetition. You have to find a comfortable position for your noggin—either down with your chin on the horizontal pad or lifted slightly up off the pad—and then maintain that position throughout the exercise.

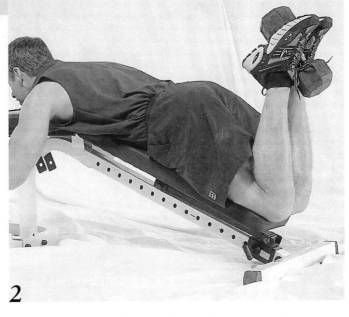

HOME VERSION

DUMBBELL LEG CURL

START

Lie on your bench and grab a dumbbell between your feet. Hold on to the bench however you can, though it's best if you can grab the bench's legs near the floor, at the end nearest your head.

1

FINISH

Slowly lift your feet toward your butt. Without pausing, slowly return to the starting position.

DO IT RIGHT

❶ Since you're not working on a machine here, the act of lifting the weight is going to be difficult only when you're working against gravity. When you get to the *2* top of the movement, there's no resistance from gravity, so don't pause there; pausing is like taking a break in the middle of each repetition.

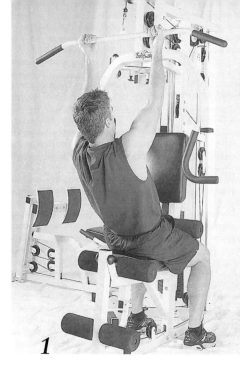

1

UNDERHAND-GRIP LAT PULLDOWN

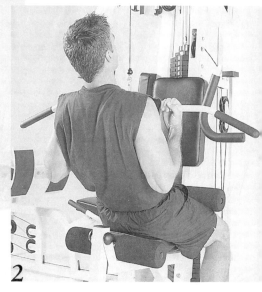

2

START

Attach a straight bar to the high pulley of the lat pulldown station. Grab the bar with an underhand, shoulder-width grip, and position yourself in the station so your upper thighs are beneath the pad. Lean back slightly, and start with a very slight bend in your elbows.

FINISH

Pull the bar to your chest, pause, then slowly return to the starting position.

DO IT RIGHT

☝ Start the set with your arms and upper body tight, and don't relax your muscles until you finish the set. The more tension you keep on your muscles, the more benefit you'll see from the exercise.

☝ Keep your upper body in a fixed position throughout the movement. If you lean back to finish a repetition, you bring your hips and lower back into the exercise, which makes it easier—and less productive—for your upper-back muscles.

ONE-ARM DUMBBELL ROW

START

Grab a dumbbell in your left hand and rest your right knee and right palm on the bench. Your left foot should be on the floor, your left knee slightly bent, and your back straight. Hold the dumbbell so your arm hangs straight down from your shoulder and your palm faces right.

1

FINISH

Lift the weight to the left side of your abdomen, with your elbow bending about 90 degrees. Pause, then slowly lower to the starting position. Finish the set, then repeat with your right arm, resting your left hand and knee on the bench.

DO IT RIGHT

☝ Focus on your back muscles: Concentrate on using them to pull your arm back to start the movement, rather than on beginning the movement with your arm.

2

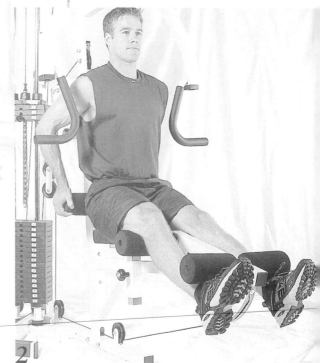

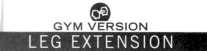
START

Sit in the leg extension machine with your back flat against the vertical pad and the leg pads against your shins, just above your feet. Bend your hips, knees, and ankles 90 degrees, forming three right angles.

FINISH

Extend your lower legs until your legs are almost straight. Pause, then slowly lower the weight to the starting position.

DO IT RIGHT

☝ You'll see some of the big guys in the gym rock forward as they do this exercise, as if they were doing a leg extension and an abdominal crunch at the same time. They're trying to squeeze out a more complete contraction in the topmost parts of their quadriceps muscles, but you don't need to worry about doing this. It's more important to make sure you keep your back against the vertical pad and concentrate on feeling a good squeeze throughout your quadriceps.

☝ If your hips lift up off the seat, you know either you're using too much weight or the seat isn't properly adjusted to your height.

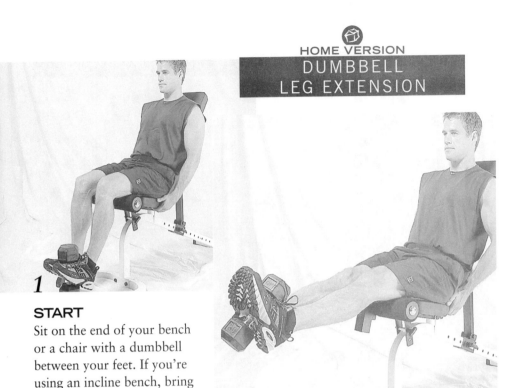

1

START

Sit on the end of your bench or a chair with a dumbbell between your feet. If you're using an incline bench, bring it up to a 75-degree angle.

2

FINISH

Extend your lower legs until your legs are almost straight. Pause, then slowly lower the weight to the starting position.

DO IT RIGHT

🛑 Your legs should go through a full 90-degree range of motion. If the angle is much smaller, you may need to use phone books to raise the bench beneath your legs.

🛑 As with the dumbbell leg curl, you have to be conscious of the fact that you're working against gravity in only part of the movement. The first part of this exercise is very easy; the movement feels hard only at the end, when your legs are nearly straight. A good strategy, therefore, is to pause in that position for 2 full seconds.

🛑 When you lower the weight all the way down, you get sort of a pendulum effect, and it's very easy to use momentum to get the weight started upward again. You can avoid that by lowering the weight only two-thirds of the way on each repetition. That way, you resist gravity on the way up and on the way down, never using momentum to assist in the lift.

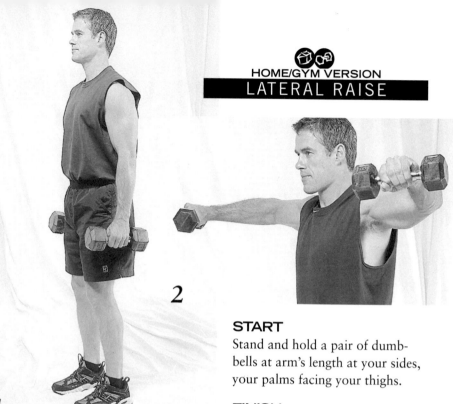

2

1

START
Stand and hold a pair of dumbbells at arm's length at your sides,
your palms facing your thighs.

FINISH
Keeping a slight bend in your el-
bows, raise the weights out to your sides until your upper arms are parallel to
the floor. Pause, then slowly return to the starting position.

DO IT RIGHT
☝ The more you bend your elbows, the more weight you can lift. But the
muscle strength you build is the same—changing your elbow angle just
changes the amount of leverage you give your shoulders.

☝ A lot of guys rock their bodies back and forth to hoist heavier weights
than their bodies are designed to lift. They look as if they were trying to start
two lawn mowers simultaneously. Keep your body steady, and let your shoulders do the work.

☝ Start the lift slowly and in full control of the weights. This part of the lift
is easy, so it's tempting to try to fling the weights upward and use momentum
to get through the part where your shoulder muscles have to work harder.

☝ You may feel a better pump in your deltoids if you lean forward slightly.
Bend forward a few degrees at the waist, and start with the weights hanging
in front of your thighs, rather than at your sides. Keep your lower back in its
natural alignment, and keep your torso at the same angle throughout the lift.

STANDING CALF RAISE

START

Stand on the balls of your feet on a step or block. Balance yourself by grabbing on to something with one hand—a handrail if you do this on the stairs at home, for example.

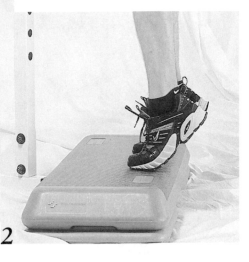

1

2

FINISH

Lower your heels as far as you can, then rise up on your toes as high as you can. Pause, feel the squeeze in your calf muscles, then repeat the full range of motion.

DO IT RIGHT

👕 You'll see guys in the gym turning their toes in and out to hit their "inner" or "outer" calves. There's no harm in doing this, but there's no point, either. Your calves work the same way whether your toes are pointed in or out. You can benefit your calf development by trying to push off on the insides of the balls of your feet, beneath your big toes. This emphasizes the inner halves of your main calf muscles, the gastrocnemii, and ensures that you work your calves evenly (as opposed to the common practice of "rolling" the weight onto the outer segments of your feet, which limits development of the inner portions of your calves and can place great strain on the lateral aspects of your ankles). But because this is a subtle move, most beginners are best off simply trying to feel a good squeeze throughout their calf muscles on each repetition and letting the shape of the muscles take care of itself.

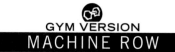
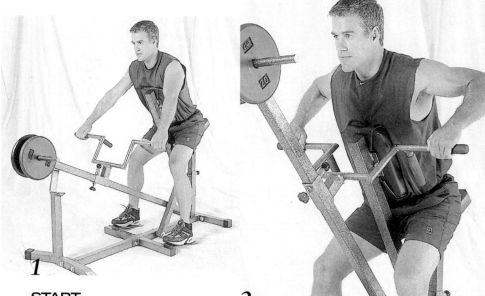

1

2

START

Position yourself in the row machine with your chest against the pad. Most machines give you two choices of handles. Grasp the ones that make your palms face the floor so the movement mirrors the chest press.

FINISH

Pull the handles back as far as you can, pause, then slowly return to the starting position.

DO IT RIGHT

🅣 Keep your torso upright throughout the exercise, with your chest forward and your lower back slightly arched.

🅣 In the finish position, you want your upper arms to be almost perpendicular to your torso. This puts the emphasis on the middle parts of your traps and rhomboids—the muscles in the middle of your back—and on your rear deltoids.

1

START

Sit on the end of your bench holding a pair of very light dumb-bells. Lean forward as *2* far as you can, and let the weights hang at arm's length. Your thumbs should be turned toward each other, and your elbows should be slightly bent.

FINISH

Slowly raise the dumbbells out to your sides as high as you can, using an arcing motion. Keep your elbows at the same angle throughout the lift. Pause at the top, feeling the squeeze in your rear-shoulder and middle-back muscles. Then slowly lower the weights to the starting position.

DO IT RIGHT

⊕ This is a "feel" exercise; it'll take a few times before you can truly tell that your rear deltoids are lifting the weight. Stick with light weights and slow repetitions, and you'll feel the muscles as they grow fatigued.

⊕ Be cautious when increasing weight. This is one of the easiest exercises to cheat on, since it feels natural to generate a little momentum with your lower torso. Next thing you know, you're flinging up much heavier weights—and hardly using your rear shoulders at all. This is a finesse exercise, designed to ensure muscle balance. It's not a powerlift.

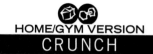

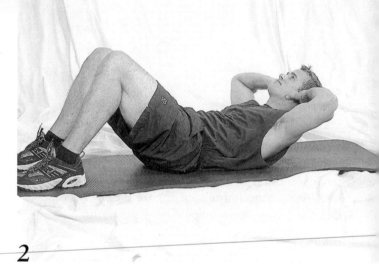

1

START

Lie on your back on the floor with your knees bent and your feet flat on the floor. Place your fingers behind your ears, with your elbows out to the sides.

FINISH *2*

Lift your shoulder blades off the floor as you crunch your rib cage toward your pelvis. Feel the squeeze in your abdominal muscles, then slowly return to the starting position.

DO IT RIGHT

☻ Although most guys consider the crunch too easy, it gets a lot harder if you do it right. Keep your feet flat on the floor and do your repetitions slowly, and you'll find it plenty challenging for these first 2 weeks of the workout plan.

☻ To prevent strain on your neck, keep a fist's distance between your chin and chest throughout the movement. An easy way to do this is to focus your eyes on one spot on the ceiling throughout the exercise. Another trick is to point your chin upward as you raise yourself off the floor.

SEATED DUMBBELL BICEPS CURL

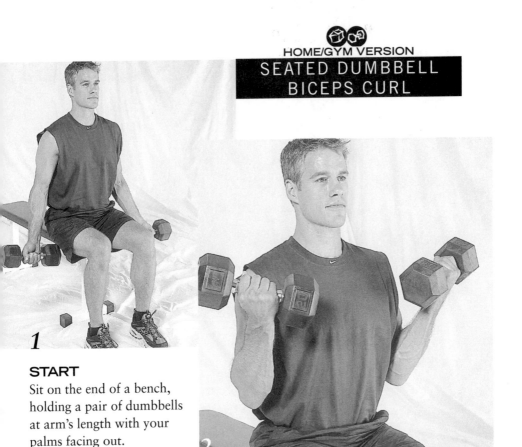

START

Sit on the end of a bench, holding a pair of dumbbells at arm's length with your palms facing out.

FINISH

Bend your elbows and slowly raise the weights as high as you can without allowing your elbows to move forward. Pause, then slowly return to the starting position.

DO IT RIGHT

❶ Keep your torso steady throughout the exercise. Rocking it back and forth adds momentum to the lift, taking work away from your biceps.

❶ This is an exercise that everyone can "feel" from the very first workout, so make the most of it. Lift slowly, keep constant tension on your biceps throughout the movement, and envision your arms growing from little-bitty hot dogs to giant Bavarian sausages.

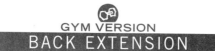
1

START
Position your-
self in the back
extension sta-
tion. Hook your
feet under the
leg anchors, and
cross your arms
over your chest.
Lower your
upper body
until your torso
is just short of
being perpendic-
ular to the floor.

2

FINISH
Raise your upper body until it is slightly above parallel to the floor. At this
point, you should have a slight arch in your back and your shoulder blades
should be pulled together in back.

DO IT RIGHT
🅣 As you progress, increase the degree of difficulty by holding your hands
behind your head and then straight out in front of your body. When that's
too easy, hold a weight against your chest as you do the movement.

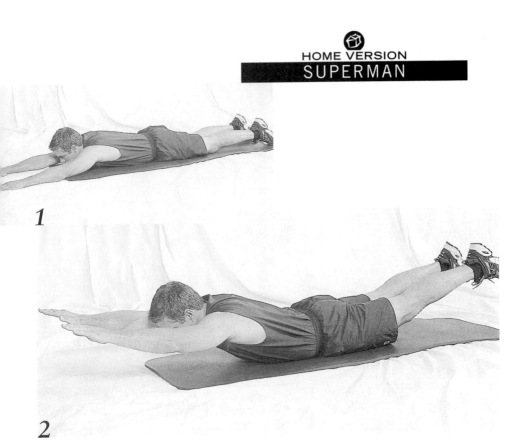

1

2

START
Lie facedown on the floor. Extend your arms out in front of you, palms down.

FINISH
Lift your arms, head, chest, thighs, and lower legs off the floor as high as possible. Hold for 3 seconds, then lower back down to the starting position.

DO IT RIGHT
🕑 You can do any number of variations to make this exercise easier, harder, or just different. You can lift only your hands and hold longer (5 to 10 seconds). You can lift one hand and the opposite leg. Most challenging? Start in a pushup position, and lift one hand and the opposite leg. When you can do more than 10 repetitions that way, you have a damn strong back.

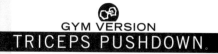
2

1

START
Attach a straight bar to a high cable. Stand in front of the machine and grab the bar with an overhand grip, your hands about shoulder-width apart and your elbows bent 90 degrees and tucked against your ribs. Place one foot in front of the other for balance, and keep your upper body in a fixed, upright position.

FINISH
Straighten your arms, keeping your elbows in close to your ribs. Pause for a second to feel the contraction in your triceps. Slowly return to the starting position.

DO IT RIGHT
❶ Keeping your upper arms in a fixed position is the key to isolating the triceps.

❶ Many people turn this simple triceps exercise into a total-body movement. The most common mistake is leaning forward, using abdominal, chest, and shoulder muscles to push the weight down. That's fine form if you're digging a ditch, but it's a lousy way to emphasize your triceps.

❶ Another common variation in form is bringing the bar up to your chin on each repetition. It's not a disaster if you allow your elbows to bend a little more than 90 degrees—you can still push the bar back down using mostly triceps—but the higher up you bring the bar, the more you involve other muscles when you push it back down again. Note: This exercise can place great strain on your elbows.

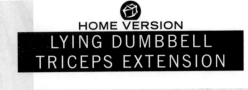

START

Grab a pair of dumbbells and
lie on your back on your bench, your feet flat on the floor. Hold the dumbbells over your head with straight arms, your palms facing each other.

FINISH

Without moving your upper arms, bend at the elbows and slowly lower the
weights as far as you can. Then raise them back to the starting position.

DO IT RIGHT

➊ As in the triceps pushdown on the previous page, the key to isolating your
triceps is keeping your upper arms in a fixed position.

➊ Many guys turn this exercise into a pullover, moving their upper arms up
toward their ears while they lower the dumbbells and then bringing them
back over their chests. Adding that movement involves your lats and chest,
making it a much less effective triceps exercise.

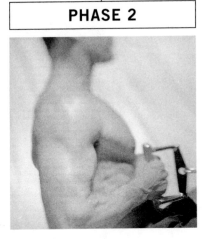

THE
TESTOSTERONE
ADVANTAGE™ WORKOUT

The Testosterone Advantage™ Workout: Phase 2

Okay, guys, we promised muscle, and now we're going to deliver muscle.

The exercises here are the weight-room classics—the presses and rows and curls—and the only goal of these workouts is to put solid muscle on your frame. That said, we aren't going to let you fling weights around mook-style. Even if your body would let you get away with it, it's not the best way to build muscle. We want you to pump them out slowly, in full control of the weight. If you want a verbal cue to keep you from hitting the accelerator halfway through the set, repeat this phrase on every repetition: "Lift weights slow, build muscle fast."

PHASE-2 GOAL: Muscle hypertrophy (muscle growth)

DURATION: 3 weeks

FREQUENCY: Three workouts per week, rotating between two different workouts. The first week, do workout A twice and workout B once. The next week, do the opposite. Ultimately, you'll have done A five times and B four.

EXERCISES: Six or eight per workout

TECHNIQUE: Supersets. Pairs of exercises are designated W-1 and

W-2, X-1 and X-2, Y-1 and Y-2, Z-1 and Z-2. Do one set of W-1, rest for 60 seconds, then do a set of W-2. Rest for 60 seconds and repeat, until you've done two or three sets each of those two exercises (how many to do is specified in the workout logs). Then move on to X-1 and X-2, and so on.

WARMUP: After a brief general warmup to raise your core temperature, use your first superset of each exercise as a more specific warmup. Use two-thirds to three-quarters of the weight you'll use in subsequent supersets, and do 8 to 10 repetitions. Never push your muscles to exhaustion on warmup sets.

REST: 60 seconds between sets

REPETITIONS: 8 to 12 per set. As soon as you hit 12 repetitions with a weight, increase the weight in the next workout.

TEMPO: Each exercise has a designated speed, listed as three numbers in the "Tempo" columns of the workout logs. Here's what those numbers mean.

First number: This is the lowering, or negative, portion of the lift. If this number is 4, that means you spend 4 seconds lowering the weight.

Second number: Pause. On most exercises, this is 1 or 2. That means you pause for 1 or 2 seconds after moving the weight. If it's 0, don't pause at all.

Third number: This is the lifting, or positive, portion of the exercise. On most exercises, this is designated as 1, which means raise the weight at your natural speed of about 1 second. If it's 2 or 3, deliberately slow down the lift and focus on feeling the muscle work. If it's X, as in the leg curl in workout B, lift the weight as fast as you can.

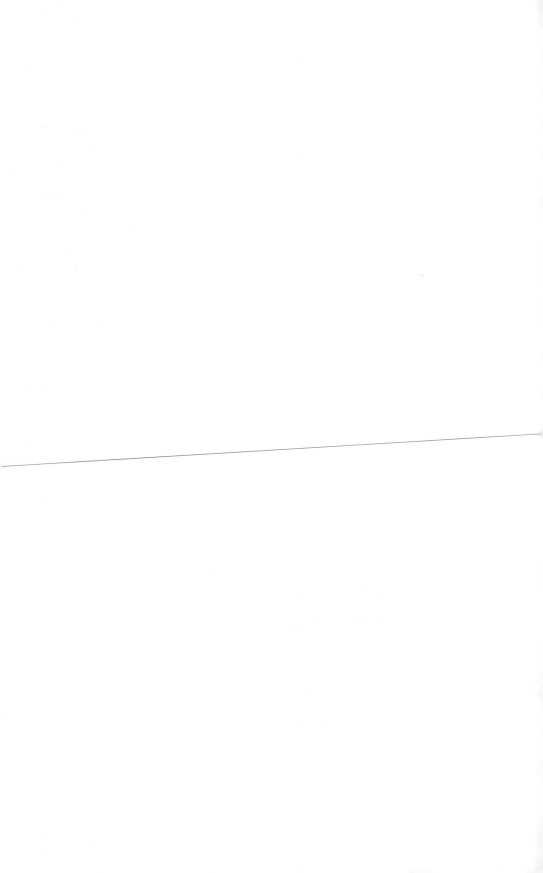

WORKOUT A

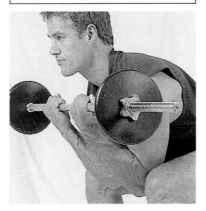

PHASE 2

Phase 2, Workout A

	TEMPO	WEEK 1 WORKOUT 1	
Barbell bench press	3-1-1	WEIGHT	REPS
Set 1			
Set 2			
Set 3			
Cable row (or one-arm dumbbell row)	2-2-2	WEIGHT	REPS
Set 1			
Set 2			
Set 3			
Lat pulldown (or reverse pushup)	4-1-1	WEIGHT	REPS
Set 1			
Set 2			
Set 3			
Barbell shoulder press	4-0-1	WEIGHT	REPS
Set 1			
Set 2			
Set 3			
Lying triceps extension with EZ bar	3-2-1	WEIGHT	REPS
Set 1			
Set 2			
Set 3 (optional)			
Preacher curl (or barbell concentration curl)	4-1-1	WEIGHT	REPS
Set 1			
Set 2			
Set 3 (optional)			
Dumbbell external rotation	3-0-3	WEIGHT	REPS
Set 1			
Set 2			
Swiss-ball crunch (or crunch with towel)	2-1-1	WEIGHT	REPS
Set 1			
Set 2			

		WEEK 2		WEEK 3			
WORKOUT 3		WORKOUT 5		WORKOUT 7		WORKOUT 9	
EIGHT	REPS	WEIGHT	REPS	WEIGHT	REPS	WEIGHT	REPS
EIGHT	REPS	WEIGHT	REPS	WEIGHT	REPS	WEIGHT	REPS
EIGHT	REPS	WEIGHT	REPS	WEIGHT	REPS	WEIGHT	REPS
EIGHT	REPS	WEIGHT	REPS	WEIGHT	REPS	WEIGHT	REPS
EIGHT	REPS	WEIGHT	REPS	WEIGHT	REPS	WEIGHT	REPS
EIGHT	REPS	WEIGHT	REPS	WEIGHT	REPS	WEIGHT	REPS
EIGHT	REPS	WEIGHT	REPS	WEIGHT	REPS	WEIGHT	REPS
EIGHT	REPS	WEIGHT	REPS	WEIGHT	REPS	WEIGHT	REPS

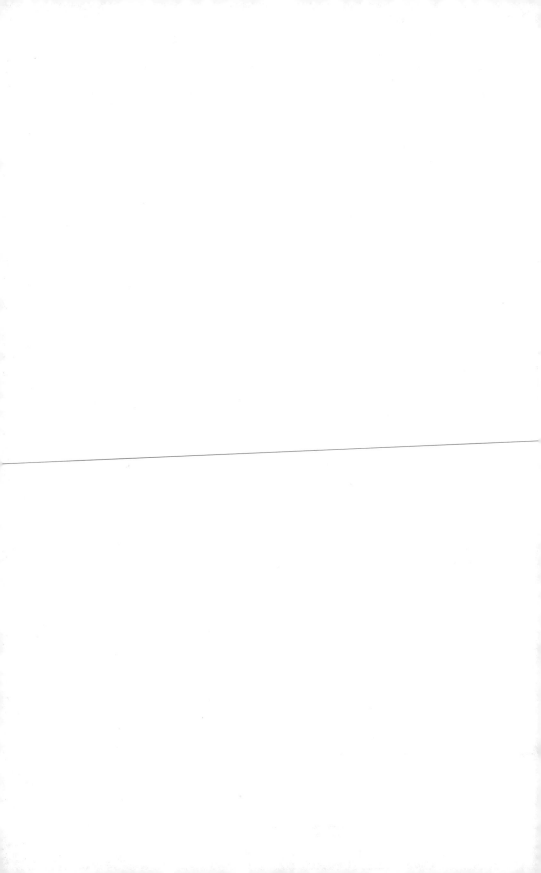

BARBELL BENCH PRESS

START

Lie on your back on a bench, feet flat on the floor. Grab the bar with your hands just wider than shoulder-width apart. Lift the bar off the uprights and hold it over your chest with your arms fully extended.

1

FINISH

Lower the bar to your chest, pause, then push it back to the starting position.

DO IT RIGHT

 The biggest cheat in bench pressing is arching *2*
your lower back so much that your butt comes off the bench. You can't completely flatten your back on this move, but you do have to keep your rear down. Lifting your butt is just a way of using gravity and momentum to push the weight up for you. And it's not too healthy for your back, either.

 Most guys regard the bench press as a straight-up-and-down movement, but in reality, the lift has a bit of an arc to it. The weight goes from your chest to just over your collarbone—hardly a straight vertical line. This is the biggest reason why doing the bench press on a Smith machine, the barbell-on-rails device found in most gyms, is not the same as doing it with a traditional barbell.

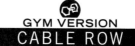

1

START

Attach a straight bar to the low cable. Sit and grab the bar with an underhand grip. Set your body with your torso upright, your shoulders back, and your arms almost straight in front of you.

2

FINISH

Pull the bar to your midsection. Pause, then slowly return to the starting position.

DO IT RIGHT

☯ This, like the bench press, is a multijoint exercise, meaning more than one joint is supposed to move. Exercises that move several joints prompt the most muscle development (and, since they're the hardest, they lead to the biggest testosterone release). But *multijoint* doesn't mean "every joint." By design, your shoulders and elbows both move, working your upper- and middle-back muscles (lats, middle traps, rear deltoids), your biceps, and your forearms. But many people in the gym—mooks, mookesses, and the misinformed—add a third move, bending and straightening at the waist as well. This adds the lower-back muscles to the exercise. There's nothing wrong with working your lower back. It's just that this isn't a particularly good way to do it. And if you insert your lower back into this exercise, you take work away from your middle and upper back since the lower-back movement adds momentum to the lift.

ONE-ARM DUMBBELL ROW

START

Grab a dumbbell in your right hand and rest your left knee and left palm on the bench. Your right foot should be on the floor, your right knee slightly bent, and your back flat. Hold a dumbbell so your arm hangs down and your palm faces left.

1

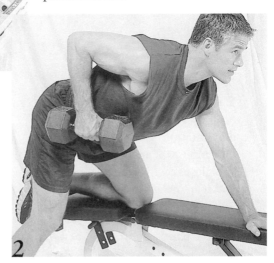

2

FINISH

Lift the weight to the right side of your abdomen, with your elbow bending about 90 degrees. Pause, then slowly lower to the starting position. Finish the set, then repeat with your left arm, resting your right hand and knee on the bench.

DO IT RIGHT

☞ If you've watched the mooks do any type of one-arm row, you've seen them rotate their torsos so their dumbbells go a little higher. Obviously, this extra twist doesn't offer any benefit to the upper-back muscles you're targeting. In fact, it takes work away from them since the twisting adds a lot of momentum to the lift. Keep your torso immobile throughout the exercise. You want to move at the shoulder and elbow joints, and nowhere else.

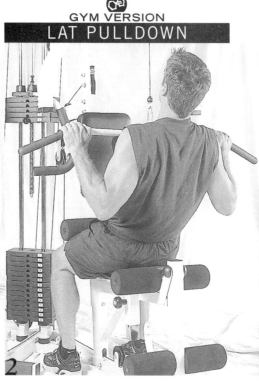

GYM VERSION
LAT PULLDOWN

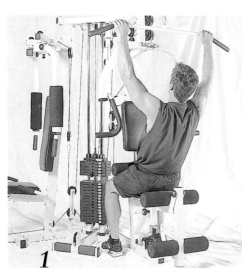

START

Position yourself in the lat pull-down station with your knees under the pad, and grab the straight bar with an overhand grip, your hands just wider than shoulder-width apart.

FINISH

Pull the bar down to your chest, pause, and slowly return to the starting position.

DO IT RIGHT

☊ You can sabotage your form in two ways: First is the mook method, in which you rise off the seat at the start of the movement, then yank your butt down and lean backward, creating momentum to get the bar to your chest.

Second is the weenie way, in which you roll your shoulders forward to finish the last rep or two, bringing the bar down in front of your chest without it actually touching you.

The best form is to slightly tilt back your head and shoulders and push up your chest to meet the bar, keeping your torso from leaning back. This position forces the strongest contraction in your lats. Leaning back recruits the trapezius more and gives the lats a slightly easier time of it.

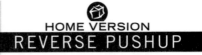

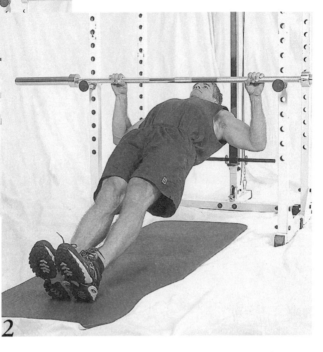

1

2

START

Attach a chinup bar in-
side a doorway, 3 to 4
feet off the floor. Grab
the bar with an over-
hand grip that's just
wider than shoulder-
width. Hang from the bar at arm's length so your body is fully extended and
only your heels rest on the floor.

FINISH

Pull yourself up as high as you can, pause, then slowly lower yourself to the
starting position.

DO IT RIGHT

☮ You probably won't be able to get your chest all the way up to the bar;
just try to get it as close as possible.

☮ Keep your body straight throughout the movement.

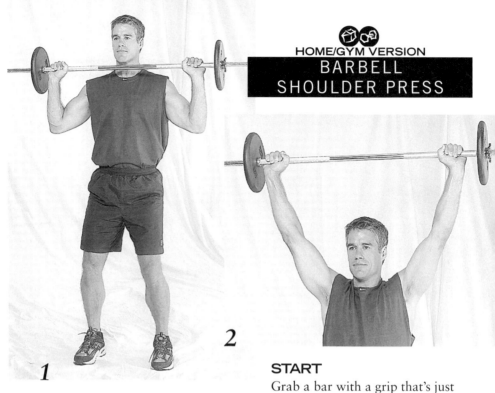

2

1

START
Grab a bar with a grip that's just wider than shoulder-width. Stand and hold the bar just above your chest.

FINISH
Push the weight up until your arms are fully extended. Don't pause. As soon as you get to the top, slowly lower back to your chest.

DO IT RIGHT
❶ Like the bench press, this isn't a straight-up-and-down lift. The bar needs to start at your chest and end up over your head, and to do that, it has to somehow get around your face. So you need to lean your head back a little at the start of the lift. Some guys, however, lean back so far that they turn the exercise into a standing chest press. Offhand, we can't think of many things that would be more dangerous to your lower back. Stay as upright as possible throughout the lift.

❶ Another great cheat is to bend your knees and straighten them as you push the weight upward. This is okay if you're training for sports by doing an exercise called the push press that is used to develop athletic power for basketball or volleyball. But for your purposes here, you want to keep your legs nearly straight. Don't lock your knees, but don't change their angle during the lift.

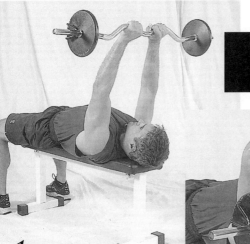

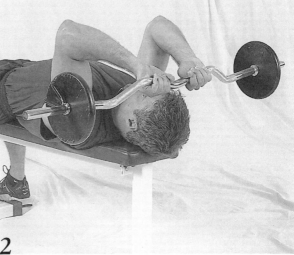

1

START
Grab an EZ-curl bar and lie back on a bench, holding the bar straight up over your chest.

FINISH

2

Slowly lower the bar to your forehead or just behind it (whichever is more comfortable), pause, then push back to the starting position.

DO IT RIGHT

🔵 Unless you've had a history of shoulder problems, we recommend that you do this movement with your upper arms angled slightly back toward your head; it makes it much more effective. But you can keep them perpendicular to your torso, if that's more comfortable for your elbows. Whichever way you choose, keep that same upper-arm position throughout the lift. That'll ensure that your triceps do all the work. Moving your upper arms on this exercise recruits your lats and chest, and there are far better ways to work those muscles.

🔵 Don't "bounce" the weight out of the bottom position. Anytime you lower a barbell near your head like this, control is important, for multiple reasons. (There's a reason why they call this exercise a skull crusher.) Even if you don't crack your head, you aren't doing your elbows any favors by using momentum to quickly lower and then raise the weight.

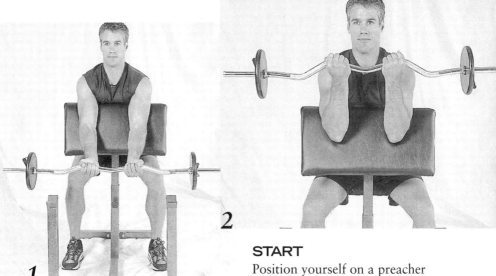

START

Position yourself on a preacher bench so that your armpits rest at the top of the pad. Grasp the EZ bar with a shoulder-width, underhand grip. Rest the backs of your upper arms on the pad and let the bar hang at arm's length.

FINISH

Curl the bar up until your hands are about 6 inches from your shoulders, pause, then lower the bar back down to the starting position.

DO IT RIGHT

🕈 The preacher bench was invented to isolate the biceps, so only your forearms should move. Keep your upper arms on the pad at all times.

🕈 If you are seated properly, you should be able to draw a straight line from your head down to your hips through the entire lift. If you shift from this position or use back muscles on the lift, you're using too much weight.

BARBELL CONCENTRATION CURL

START

Grab a barbell with a narrow underhand grip, your hands 4 to 6 inches apart. Sit on the end of your bench with your feet about 12 inches apart, and lean forward until your upper body is nearly parallel to the floor. Your elbows should touch the insides of your knees but not rest on them. Allow your arms to hang down toward the floor.

1

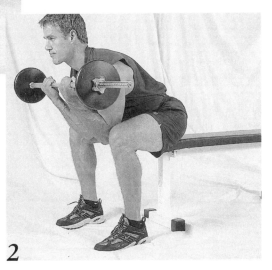

2

FINISH

Slowly curl the bar up toward your chin, keeping your upper arms stationary. Pause, then slowly lower back to the starting position.

DO IT RIGHT

🍏 The concentration curl is aptly named; if you're doing it right, you should be fully focused on how your biceps feel throughout each repetition.

🍏 Keep your elbows in contact with your knees throughout the exercise.

🍏 Keep your head in line with your torso. Maintain this head and torso position throughout the exercise.

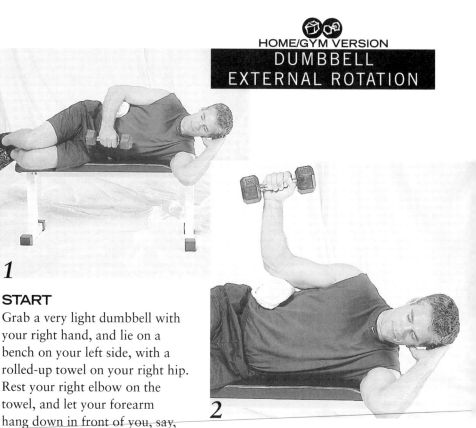

DUMBBELL EXTERNAL ROTATION

1

START

Grab a very light dumbbell with your right hand, and lie on a bench on your left side, with a rolled-up towel on your right hip. Rest your right elbow on the towel, and let your forearm hang down in front of you, say,

2

a couple of inches in front of your abdomen. Keep your right wrist straight.

FINISH

Slowly raise your forearm as high as you can by rotating your upper arm. Don't pause. Slowly lower the weight. Finish the set with your right arm, then switch positions and repeat with your left arm.

DO IT RIGHT

ⓣ There aren't any bragging rights bestowed upon the guy with the strongest rotator cuffs. The only satisfaction you'll gain is when you lift longer than the guys who neglect these crucial and easily injured muscles. (Although the internal rotators are involved in more athletic motions, especially throwing, the external rotators are the most frequently injured in the weight room, often because of an imbalance between muscles on the front of the body and those on the back. Overenthusiastic bench pressing or underenthusiastic rowing can create this imbalance in a hurry.) So select a very light weight to start—a 5-pound dumbbell will work for most guys—and focus on slowly working your arm through the full range of motion.

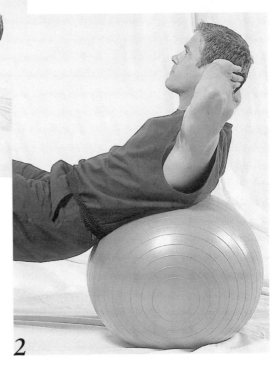

1

START
Lie on your back on a Swiss ball, fingers behind your ears.

FINISH
Raise your head and shoulders and crunch your rib cage toward your pelvis. Pause, and slowly return to the starting position.

2

DO IT RIGHT

🔻 The reason for doing a crunch on a ball instead of on the floor is to add about 30 degrees to your range of motion. That makes the muscles in your rectus abdominis work harder and thus grow more. So the only real way to cheat yourself on this exercise is to shorten your range of motion.

🔻 A second benefit of the exercise is that the ball puts your body on an unstable surface, so other muscles in your trunk and lower body—obliques, gluteals, thighs—have to do some work to keep you balanced throughout the exercise.

🔻 When you can finish 12 repetitions in both sets, add resistance. Hold a weight plate or dumbbell under your chin. Then, in subsequent workouts, progressively add more weight.

HOME
VERSION
ON NEXT PAGE

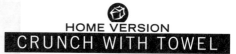
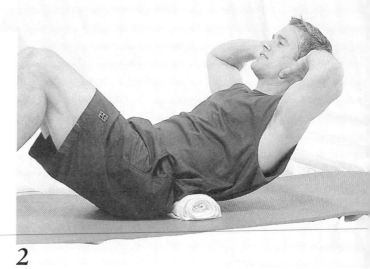

START

Lie on your back on the floor, with a rolled-up towel in the small of your back. Place your fingers behind your ears.

1

FINISH

Crunch your rib cage toward your pelvis as you lift your head and shoulders off the floor. Pause, then slowly return to the starting position.

2

DO IT RIGHT

☻ The towel propping up your lower back will add some range of motion to this exercise, but it still won't feel a whole lot different from the crunch you did in phase 1. So you'll probably need to add weight. Hold a weight plate or dumbbell under your chin. Added weight can mean added stress on your neck, so it's even more important to keep a fist's distance between your chin and chest.

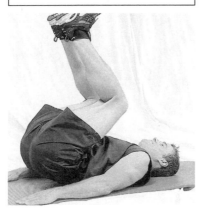

PHASE 2

Phase 2, Workout B

	TEMPO	WEEK 1 WORKOUT 2	
x1 Leg press (or split squat)	4-2-1	WEIGHT	REPS
Set 1			
Set 2			
Set 3			
x2 Leg curl (or dumbbell leg curl)	5-1-X	WEIGHT	REPS
Set 1			
Set 2			
Set 3			
y1 Leg extension (or dumbbell leg extension)	2-0-2	WEIGHT	REPS
Set 1			
Set 2			
Set 3			
y2 Back extension (or Superman)	3-1-1	WEIGHT	REPS
Set 1			
Set 2			
Set 3			
z1 Seated calf raise (or free-weight seated calf raise)	2-0-2	WEIGHT	REPS
Set 1			
Set 2			
Set 3 (optional)			
z2 Reverse crunch	4-1-1	WEIGHT	REPS
Set 1			
Set 2			
Set 3 (optional)			

WEEK 2				WEEK 3	
WORKOUT 4		WORKOUT 6		WORKOUT 8	
WEIGHT	REPS	WEIGHT	REPS	WEIGHT	REPS
WEIGHT	REPS	WEIGHT	REPS	WEIGHT	REPS
WEIGHT	REPS	WEIGHT	REPS	WEIGHT	REPS
WEIGHT	REPS	WEIGHT	REPS	WEIGHT	REPS
WEIGHT	REPS	WEIGHT	REPS	WEIGHT	REPS
WEIGHT	REPS	WEIGHT	REPS	WEIGHT	REPS

WORKOUT B STARTS WITH FOUR EXERCISES THAT YOU LEARNED IN PHASE 1.

GYM VERSION
LEG PRESS

HOME VERSION
SPLIT SQUAT

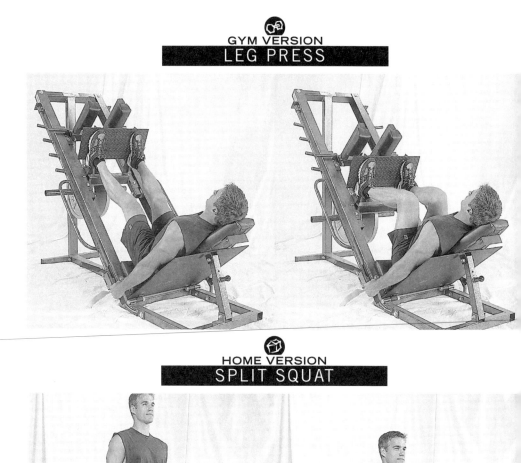

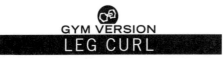

GYM VERSION
LEG CURL

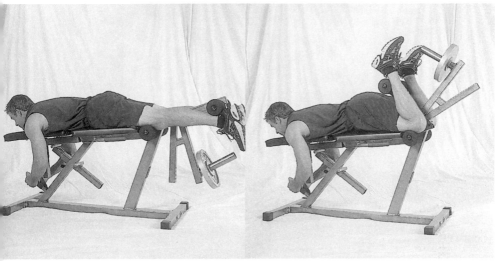

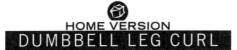

HOME VERSION
DUMBBELL LEG CURL

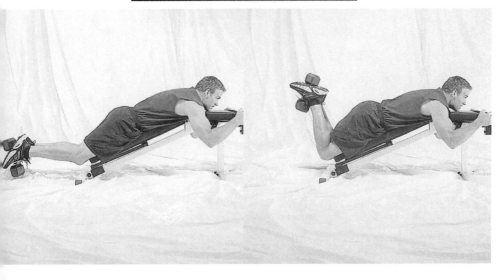

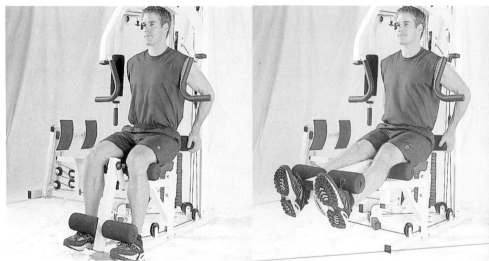

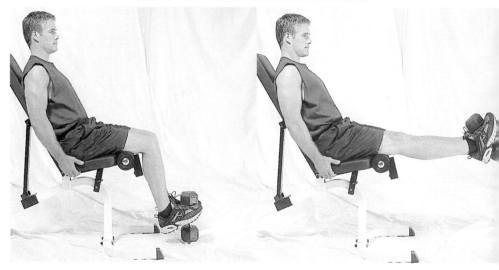

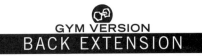

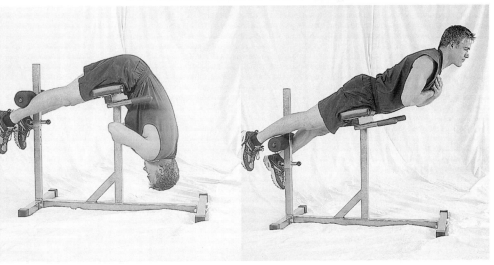

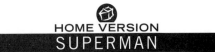

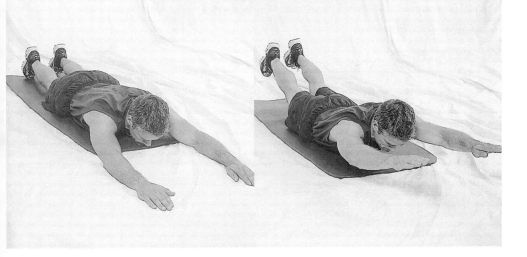

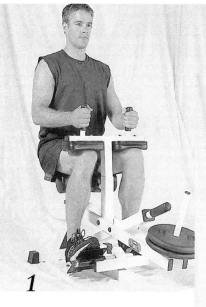

1

START
Sit in the seated calf raise machine with the balls of your feet on the platform and the pad across your lower thighs. Release the support, and lower your heels as far as you can.

FINISH

2

Lift your heels as high as you can. Without pausing, lower them to the starting position.

DO IT RIGHT
☝ Even in a no-bragging-rights exercise like the seated calf raise, you see guys cheating, usually by pulling up on the pads with their hands. Hey, it's a calf exercise—let your calves do the work. Keep your hands to your sides if you can't resist the urge to use them in the exercise. It's not as if you'd fall off the machine if you didn't hold on.

FREE-WEIGHT SEATED CALF RAISE

START

Sit on the end of your bench with the balls of your feet on a small platform (even a two-by-four will do). Let your heels hang over the edge. Rest a barbell across your lower thighs, just above your knees, or hold a dumbbell in the same spot on each leg. Lower your heels as far as you can.

1

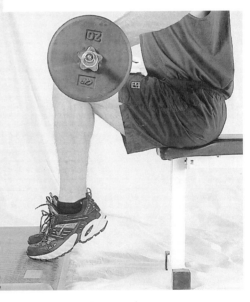

2

FINISH

Lift your heels as high as you can. Without pausing, lower them to the starting position.

DO IT RIGHT

♆ Don't be brave; make this exercise comfortable for yourself. There's no shame in providing some padding beneath the barbell by covering your knees with a towel or even a blanket. You don't get extra points—or extra muscle—for adding bruises to your legs.

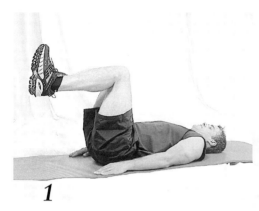

1

START
Lie on your back on the floor with your hands at your sides, palms down. Bend your hips and knees at 90-degree angles so your thighs

2

are perpendicular to the floor and your lower legs are parallel to the floor.

FINISH
Lift your hips off the floor and crunch your pelvis toward your rib cage. Pause when your abs feel fully contracted, then slowly return to the starting position.

DO IT RIGHT
⊕ This is another "feel" exercise. It may take several sets or even several workouts before you figure out the perfect range of motion. Here's a trick that may help you get it right: Imagine that your hips are a bucket of water that you're trying to empty. You're trying to lift the bucket and tilt it over.

⊕ If you've done a lot of abdominal exercises, you'll probably find it easy to do 12 repetitions of this exercise, even with perfect form and tempo. So, if you have access to one, feel free to use a slant board, with your head at the higher end. The higher the slope, the harder the exercise will be.

If you don't have a slant board, try holding a dumbbell between your feet or a medicine ball between your knees.

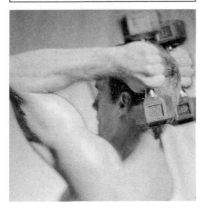

THE
TESTOSTERONE
ADVANTAGE™ WORKOUT

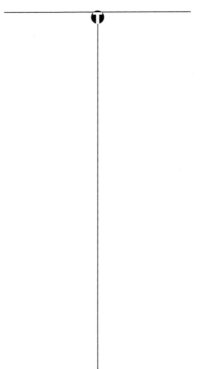

The
Testosterone Advantage™ Workout:
Phase 3

*F*or 5 weeks now, the big T dog has paced about in his pen, waiting for his opportunity to jump out and do what T dogs do: make you a stronger, more confident guy—a guy's guy. For the next 4 weeks, you'll do the hardest strength-building exercises: deadlifts, squats, presses, rows. Your body will respond by opening the spigot and letting the testosterone flow.

Warn the women and children: The juice is loose.

PHASE-3 GOAL: Strength and testosterone release

DURATION: 4 weeks

FREQUENCY: Perform each of the three workouts (designated workout A, workout B, and workout C) once a week.

EXERCISES: Four per workout

TECHNIQUE: Straight sets. Do all the sets of one exercise before moving on to the next.

WARMUP: After a brief general warmup to raise your core temperature, use the first set of each exercise as a more specific warmup. Use two-thirds to three-quarters of the weight you'll use in subsequent sets, and do five to seven repetitions. Never push your muscles to exhaustion on warmup sets.

REST: 3 minutes between sets

REPETITIONS: Four to six per set. As soon as you hit six repetitions with a weight, increase the weight in the next workout. Exceptions are exercises for abs and calves, for which you use sets of eight reps.

TEMPO: As in phase 2, each portion of an exercise has a designated speed. On many of the exercises, the actual lifting portion of the exercise is denoted by the letter X, meaning you should lift as fast as you can. Since you're using heavy weights, you don't actually fling barbells and dumbbells around. Rather, you *try* to lift them fast, pause (if the exercise calls for a pause), then lower them at the designated speed of 2, 3, or 4 seconds.

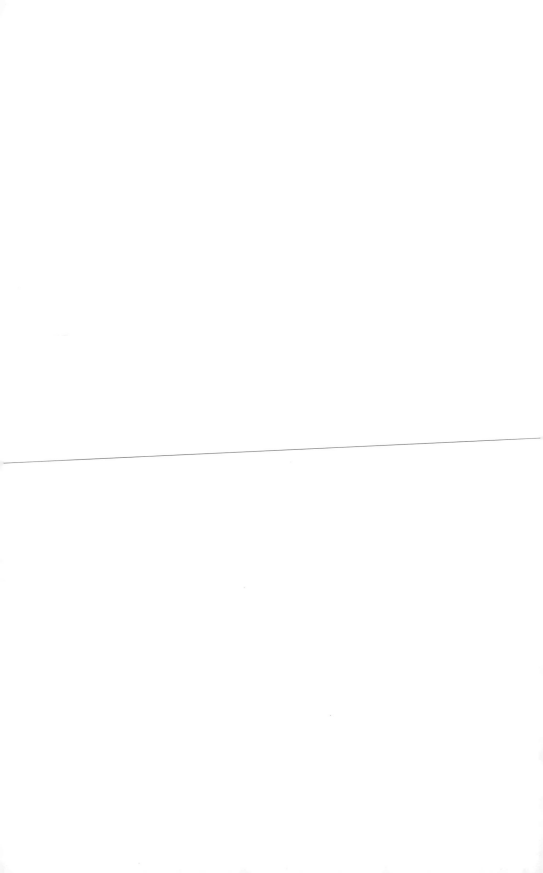

WORKOUT A

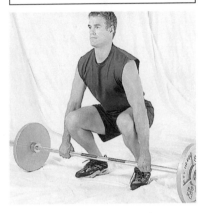

PHASE 3

Phase 3, Workout A

		TEMPO	WEEK 1 DAY 1	
			WEIGHT	REPS
1	**Deadlift**	3-1-X	WEIGHT	REPS
	Set 1			
	Set 2			
	Set 3			
	Set 4			
	Set 5			
2	**Barbell bench press**	4-1-X	WEIGHT	REPS
	Set 1			
	Set 2			
	Set 3			
	Set 4			
	Set 5			
3	**One-arm row (elbow out)**	3-1-X	WEIGHT	REPS
	Set 1			
	Set 2			
	Set 3			
	Set 4			
4	**Seated leg curl (or hip extension)**	2-2-X	WEIGHT	REPS
	Set 1			
	Set 2			
	Set 3			

WEEK 2		WEEK 3		WEEK 4	
DAY 1		DAY 1		DAY 1	
WEIGHT	REPS	WEIGHT	REPS	WEIGHT	REPS
WEIGHT	REPS	WEIGHT	REPS	WEIGHT	REPS
WEIGHT	REPS	WEIGHT	REPS	WEIGHT	REPS
WEIGHT	REPS	WEIGHT	REPS	WEIGHT	REPS

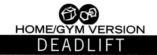
1

START

Stand with your feet shoulder-width apart. Roll a barbell against your lower legs, and grip it with your arms just outside your thighs. Bend your knees and push your butt back; you want your lower legs almost perpendicular to the floor so the lift will be straight up, rather than back and then up. Lift your head and shoulders so your eyes are **2** focused straight ahead and your shoulder blades are pulled together in back. Your lower back should be either flat or slightly arched—if it's rounded, you'll start the lift with your lower back in its weakest position, which is pretty much begging for an injury. Take a deep breath.

FINISH

Stand with the weight. Once the bar gets past your knees, exhale forcefully and drive your hips forward (picture your favorite prison movie here). Keep your shoulder blades back throughout the movement. Lower the weight carefully, keeping it as close to your shins as you can.

DO IT RIGHT

☝ A lot of the big guys in the gym use a "mixed grip"—one hand under and one hand over. We don't recommend this; you'll tend to pull the bar harder with the arm using the underhand grip (the biceps will naturally try to help out), and that can lead to uneven torque on your back. This sets you up for overuse injuries.

BARBELL BENCH PRESS

START

Lie on your back on a bench, feet flat on the floor. Grab the bar with your hands just wider than shoulder-width apart. Lift the bar off the uprights and hold it over your chest with your arms fully extended.

1

FINISH

Lower the bar to your chest, pause, then push it back to the starting position.

DO IT RIGHT

☮ Remember to keep your back flat on the bench throughout the exercise.

☮ If you train in a gym, you'll see a lot of guys doing this exercise in the Smith machine, a barbell-on-rails device. Using a machine takes away the balance component, meaning your body doesn't have to work as hard. Also, the bar itself doesn't weigh as much as a 45-pound Olympic bar, even though it looks similar. The machine is counterbalanced, so the bar may actually weigh as little as 15 pounds—what good does that do?

ONE-ARM ROW (ELBOW OUT)

START

Grab a dumbbell in your right hand, and rest your left knee and left palm on a bench. Keep your right foot on the floor, your right knee slightly bent, and your back straight. Hold the dumbbell so your arm hangs straight down from your shoulder and your knuckles point forward.

FINISH

Lift the weight so your upper arm goes out to your side, nearly perpendicular to your torso, and your elbow bends 90 degrees. Pause, then slowly lower to the starting position. Finish the set, then repeat with your left arm, resting your right hand and knee on the bench.

DO IT RIGHT

🔱 This is a distinctly different exercise from the one-arm row you've seen the mooks perform. Because your elbow is out, rather than next to your torso, you use your trapezius and rear deltoids more and your lats less. You have to use less weight than you would on the standard row.

🔱 Keep your torso still throughout the exercise. You want to move at the shoulder and elbow joints, and nowhere else.

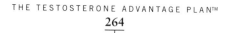

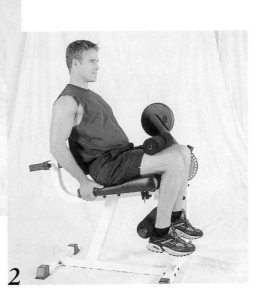

1

2

START

Sit in the seated leg curl machine with the near pad over your knees and the far pad above your heels and below your calf muscles (at the Achilles tendon, usually).

FINISH

Bend your knees and push down the far pad as low as you can. Pause, then slowly allow the pad to rise to the starting position.

DO IT RIGHT

🕦 The machine dictates form and range of motion. About the only way to screw up the exercise is to lift your hips up and down in the seat, adding momentum to the lift. The fix is simple: Sit your ass down, and keep it down.

HOME
VERSION
ON NEXT PAGE

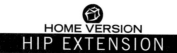
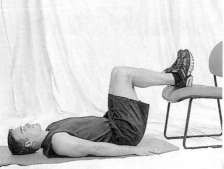

1

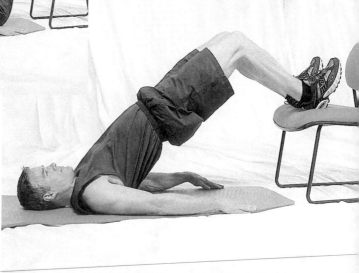

START

Lie on the floor with both heels resting on the edge of a chair or bench. (A chair is preferable; you want some extra height here.) Bend your knees 90 degrees.

2

Keep your hands on the floor at your sides, palms down. Also keep your back flat on the floor.

FINISH

Contract your hamstrings and lift your hips off the floor so your body forms a straight line from your chest to your knees. Pause, then slowly lower yourself to the starting position.

DO IT RIGHT

☝ You'll have to experiment to find a knee angle that gives your hamstrings the best challenge for five repetitions. The straighter your legs, the harder the exercise.

☝ If you have some experience lifting weights, you have to make the exercise even harder. Lift one leg directly over your hip so it's straight and perpendicular to the floor.

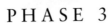

WORKOUT B

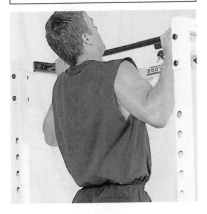

PHASE 3

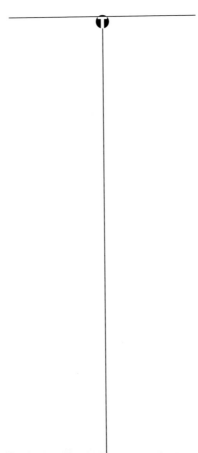

Phase 3, Workout B

	TEMPO	WEEK 1 DAY 2	
Wide-grip lat pulldown (or assisted pullup)	4-1-1	WEIGHT	REPS
Set 1			
Set 2			
Set 3			
Set 4			
Set 5			
Dumbbell stepup	2-1-X	WEIGHT	REPS
Set 1			
Set 2			
Set 3			
Set 4			
Set 5			
Overhead triceps extension	3-1-1	WEIGHT	REPS
Set 1			
Set 2			
Set 3			
Set 4			
One-legged standing calf raise	2-1-X	WEIGHT	REPS
Set 1			
Set 2			
Set 3			

WEEK 2 DAY 2		WEEK 3 DAY 2		WEEK 4 DAY 2	
WEIGHT	REPS	WEIGHT	REPS	WEIGHT	REPS
WEIGHT	REPS	WEIGHT	REPS	WEIGHT	REPS
WEIGHT	REPS	WEIGHT	REPS	WEIGHT	REPS
WEIGHT	REPS	WEIGHT	REPS	WEIGHT	REPS

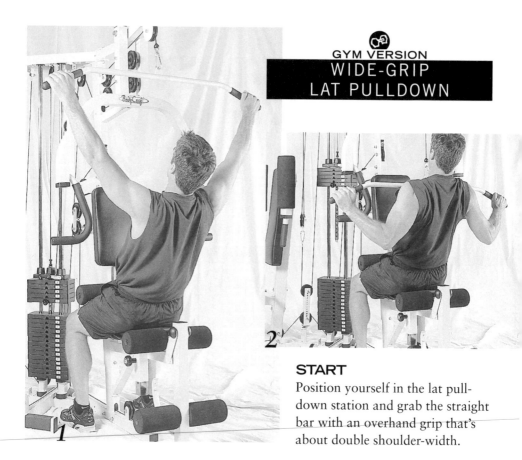

START

Position yourself in the lat pull-down station and grab the straight bar with an overhand grip that's about double shoulder-width.

FINISH

Pull the bar to your chest, pause, and slowly return to the starting position.

DO IT RIGHT

🛈 If you were tempted to cheat in phase 2, when you were doing 12-repetition sets of the lat pulldown with a shoulder-width grip, it's going to be really tough to move even heavier weights. Keep your form strict: Pull your shoulder blades back at the start of the first repetition, and try to keep them back throughout the set. It's hard to do, but it helps you feel your lats working, which keeps you focused on performing the exercise correctly.

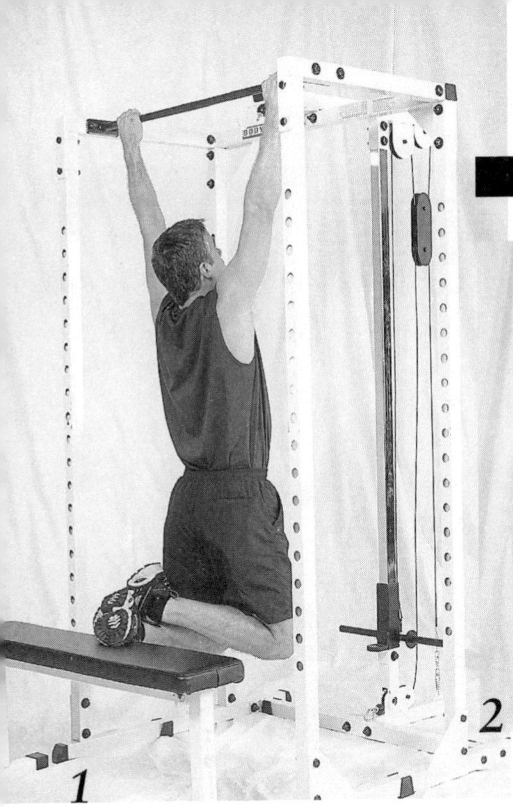

1

HOME VERSION

ASSISTED PULLUP

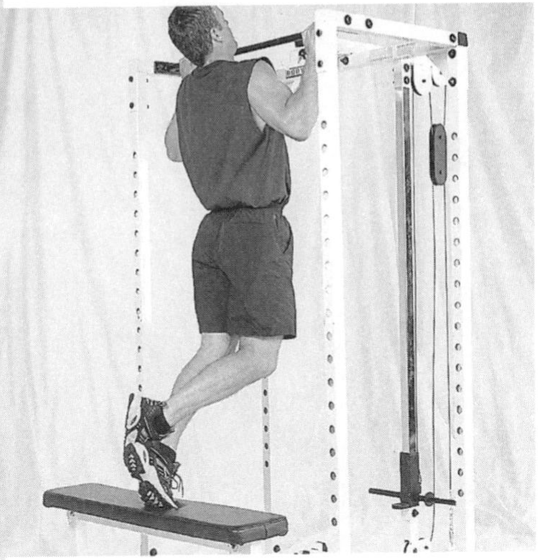

2

START

Set a bench or footstool underneath a chinup bar. Grab the bar with the widest possible overhand grip, cross your feet behind you, and rest the toes of one foot on the bench. Hang from the bar with your arms completely extended.

FINISH

Pull yourself up as high as you can. If you can't pull your entire body weight up, assist yourself by pushing up slightly with your feet. Pause, then slowly lower yourself back to the starting position.

DO IT RIGHT

- Most people who work out can't do a single pullup, so don't feel bad if you're in the majority. There are two keys to getting the full benefit of this exercise: First, force your upper body to do as much of the work as possible, using your feet as little as possible. Second, take a full 4 seconds to lower your body on each repetition.

- Try to do one more unassisted pullup in each set of each workout. So if you can do only one unassisted pullup per set the first time you do this workout, try for two per set in the second workout, three in the third, four in the fourth. That's incredibly ambitious, but if you can get to that point, you'll make your home workouts far more productive because you'll be adding the best lat-building exercise of them all to your repertoire.

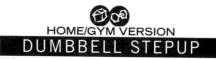

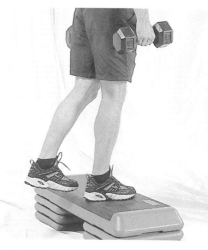

2

1

START
Grab a pair of dumbbells and stand in front of a step or bench that's 12 to 18 inches high.

FINISH
Step up onto the step with your right foot, and push off with that foot to lift the rest of your body onto the step. Step down with your left foot first, then with your right. Finish the set with your right leg, then repeat the set with your left leg, stepping up with your left and stepping down on your right.

DO IT RIGHT

◑ The key to this exercise is pushing off with the heel of the foot that's stepping up. That activates the big gluteal and hamstring muscles in that leg. If you push off with your trailing foot—the one on the floor—you use the calf muscles in that leg and take work away from the leg you're targeting.

◑ A lot of guys find they can use a lot of weight on this exercise when doing sets of 5 repetitions. Unfortunately, some of those guys may also find that it's hard to hold heavy dumbbells at arm's length. If you're one of them, it's okay to use a barbell across your shoulders. The balance is difficult to master, but the reward is that you can probably use more weight and give your lower-body muscles a more intense workout.

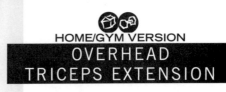

OVERHEAD TRICEPS EXTENSION

START

Grab a pair of dumbbells and sit on a bench. Raise the dumbbells straight overhead so your palms face each other.

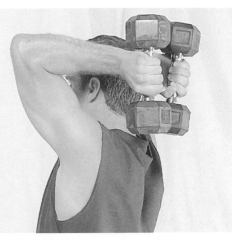

1

2

FINISH

Without moving your upper arms, bend your elbows to slowly lower the weights behind your head. Pause, then raise back to the starting position.

DO IT RIGHT

🔵 Triceps are easy muscles to work since you can actually feel them in action. But the fact that you feel them doesn't mean you're working them with good form. The key is to move only at the elbow joint; once your upper arms move forward, back, or to the sides, you've engaged other muscles.

🔵 This version—two dumbbells, neutral hand position—is probably the most elbow-friendly of all the variations on the overhead triceps extension (also called a French press). But you still need to do the exercise slowly and carefully, particularly when you lower the weights behind your head. Dropping them quickly and snapping them back up is begging for a sprained elbow ligament.

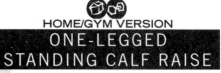
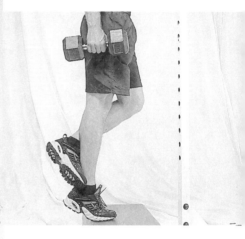

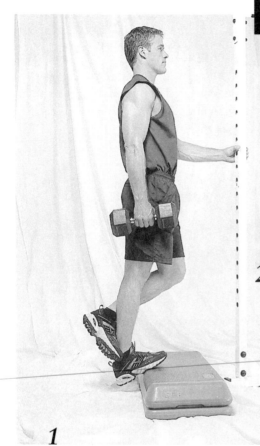

START

Grab a dumbbell in your right hand and stand on a step or block. Balance by using your left hand to hold on to whatever is nearby. Cross your left foot behind your right ankle, and balance yourself on the ball of your right foot.

FINISH

Lower your right heel as far as you can, pause, then raise as high as you can. Finish the set with your right leg, then repeat with your left.

DO IT RIGHT

❶ Although this is probably the most intense calf exercise you can do, you won't see many big guys doing it. Why not? Because you can't use as much weight when you work one leg at a time. In other words, this isn't an ego exercise. Use as much weight as you can while still getting eight great contractions in each set. But don't worry about whether the weight you're holding looks impressive. Be satisfied knowing your results will be impressive.

❶ If you work out in a gym, you can do this exercise in a standing calf raise machine. Do everything exactly the same, without holding a dumbbell.

WORKOUT C

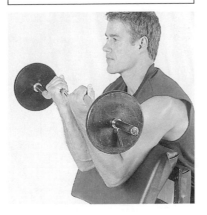

PHASE 3

Phase 3, Workout C

	TEMPO	WEEK 1 DAY 3	
		WEIGHT	REPS
Squat	3-1-1		
Set 1			
Set 2			
Set 3			
Set 4			
Set 5			
Military press	2-2-X	WEIGHT	REPS
Set 1			
Set 2			
Set 3			
Set 4			
Set 5			
Preacher curl (or barbell concentration curl)	4-0-X	WEIGHT	REPS
Set 1			
Set 2			
Set 3			
Set 4			
Incline reverse crunch (or dumbbell reverse crunch)	3-1-1	WEIGHT	REPS
Set 1			
Set 2			
Set 3			

WEEK 2		WEEK 3		WEEK 4	
DAY 3		DAY 3		DAY 3	
WEIGHT	REPS	WEIGHT	REPS	WEIGHT	REPS
WEIGHT	REPS	WEIGHT	REPS	WEIGHT	REPS
WEIGHT	REPS	WEIGHT	REPS	WEIGHT	REPS
WEIGHT	REPS	WEIGHT	REPS	WEIGHT	REPS

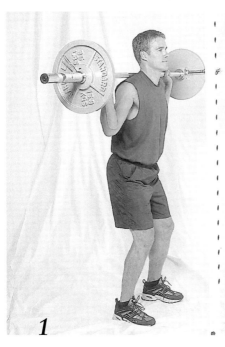

1

START
Place a barbell across your shoulders and step back from the squat rack. Set your feet shoulder-width apart, and place your hands just beyond shoulder-width apart on the bar.

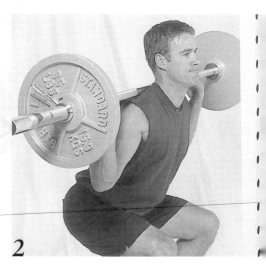

2

FINISH
Bend at the knees and hips, as if you were sitting down in a chair, and lower your body until your thighs are parallel to the floor. Pause, then rise to the starting position.

DO IT RIGHT
❂ No matter how little weight you have to use, get the range of motion correct first. You'll be able to increase weight rapidly once your body knows how to do the exercise.

❂ Ideally, your lower legs should remain close to perpendicular to the floor throughout the exercise. Conventional wisdom says your knees should never extend past your toes during this exercise. There isn't really any evidence to support this advice, but your knees will probably feel better when you adhere to it.

❂ Keep your lower back slightly arched. Bend forward as little as possible. To make this easier, point your elbows toward your thighs in the starting position, and try to keep them there. If you can touch your elbows to the outsides of your thighs in the bottom position, you're keeping your back upright *and* going through a full range of motion.

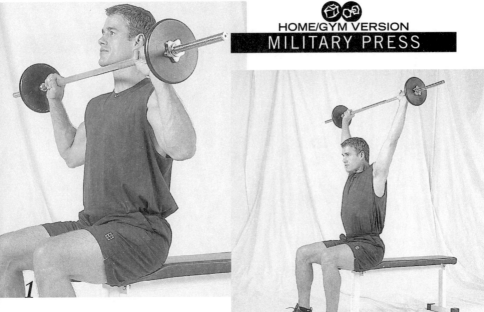

START

Grab a barbell and sit on a bench. Hold the bar at shoulder level, with your palms facing forward.

FINISH

Press the bar up until your arms are almost fully extended (don't lock your elbows or lift your shoulder blades to add an extra inch or two to your range of motion). Lower the bar, pause, and repeat.

DO IT RIGHT

🛈 Some trainers recommend that you sit with your back fully supported while doing this exercise. That makes sense if you have a history of back problems, since there is some spinal compression when you lift weights overhead. But most guys use back support just so they can push heavier weights. We think it's better to sit without support, unless you have an existing orthopedic problem. It means using less weight, but you'll develop better overall strength throughout your back and midsection if you have to hold your body upright throughout the exercise.

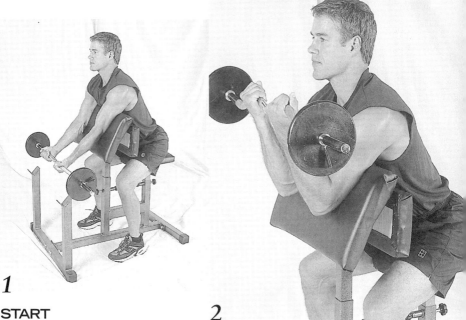

1

2

START
Position yourself on a preacher bench so that your armpits rest at the top of the pad. Grasp an EZ bar with a shoulder-width, underhand grip. Rest the backs of your upper arms on the pad and let the bar hang at arm's length.

FINISH
Curl the bar up until your hands are about 6 inches from your shoulders. Without pausing, lower the bar back down to the starting position.

DO IT BETTER
⊕ Keep constant tension on your biceps. After you lift the weight to a certain point—usually if you bend your elbows to an angle that's smaller than 90 degrees—you aren't working against gravity anymore, and your muscles don't have to work much to hold the weight. Stop the lift before you reach that point.

⊕ This is a favorite exercise among mooks, who put their upper bodies through all sorts of contortions to lift heavier weights. Ignore the impulse to pile on the plates; use only as much weight as you can handle with perfect form for all your repetitions.

1

2

START

Grab a barbell with a narrow underhand grip, your hands 4 to 6 inches apart. Sit on the end of your bench with your feet about 12 inches apart, and lean forward until your upper body is nearly parallel to the floor. Your elbows should touch the insides of your knees but not rest on them. Allow your arms to hang down toward the floor.

FINISH

Slowly curl the bar up toward your chin, keeping your upper arms stationary. Pause, then slowly lower back to the starting position.

DO IT RIGHT

☝ As you start increasing the weight you use on this exercise, you'll be tempted to lean back to finish your repetitions. Don't give in to temptation— that just takes work away from your biceps.

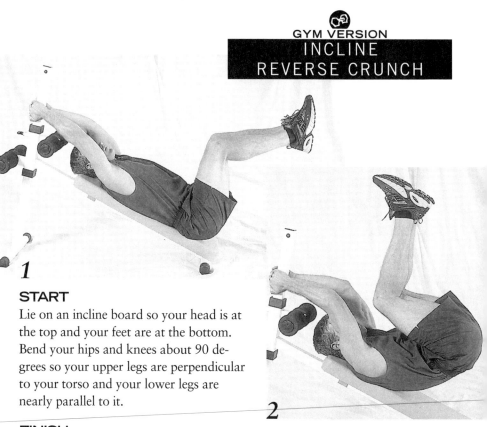

1

START

Lie on an incline board so your head is at the top and your feet are at the bottom. Bend your hips and knees about 90 degrees so your upper legs are perpendicular to your torso and your lower legs are nearly parallel to it.

2

FINISH

Lift up your hips and tilt them toward your rib cage. Pause, then slowly lower yourself to the starting position.

DO IT RIGHT

� If it's too easy to do eight repetitions, you need to add resistance. Try holding a medicine ball between your knees or a dumbbell between your feet.

� A second option is to extend your legs straight out in the starting position and then bend your knees and hips as you lift them up. This brings your hip flexors into play and can be very tough on your lower back. But if you can keep your back from arching excessively while extending your legs, you probably won't have problems with it, and you'll find it a challenging alternative.

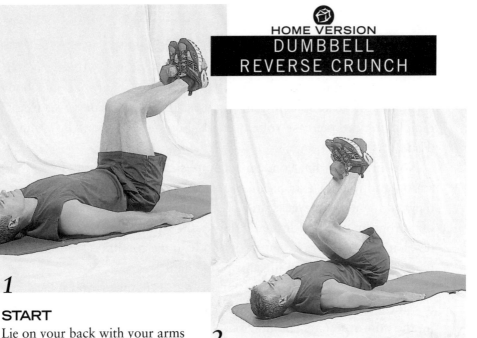

DUMBBELL REVERSE CRUNCH

1

2

START

Lie on your back with your arms against your body and your hips and knees bent 90 degrees so your upper legs are perpendicular to your torso and your lower legs are nearly parallel to it. Hold a dumbbell between your feet.

FINISH

Lift up your hips and tilt them toward your rib cage. Pause, then slowly lower yourself to the starting position.

DO IT RIGHT

☝ You can also extend your arms out to the sides if that makes it easier for you to stay balanced.

YOU'VE ONLY JUST BEGUN

The really cool thing about finishing the 9-week T workout is that you've only begun to tap the possibilities. You've seen what your body is capable of accomplishing in just over 2 months. You've seen how rapidly you can increase your strength, burn fat, and build lean muscle tissue.

Now imagine what you can accomplish with a lifetime of good nutrition and regular exercise. The results won't always come as fast as they did these past 9 weeks. In fact, the better shape you're in at the start of a program, the less dramatic the results will be. That's actually good news; it means you're keeping your body in the condition that nature intended and that modern life conspires against.

That said, *less dramatic* doesn't mean "negligible." And it certainly doesn't mean "less satisfying." You'll continue to marvel at, and revel in, the improvements you make in the months and years ahead.

In the next chapter, we'll show you how to continue your exercise odyssey beyond the T program, getting stronger, leaner, and more muscular for as long as you're willing to put in the work and celebrate the results.

Life at the Top

One of the most dreaded words in the gym lexicon is *plateau*. One of the most treasured sensations in sports—or, indeed, any pursuit—is reaching a peak. What's the difference?

A plateau is what happens when you try to stay on a peak. (Please, no flack from geography buffs; this is a fitness book, not an atlas.) You stop making progress and suddenly find yourself stranded.

Let us explain: When a mountain climber reaches a peak, he celebrates. He plants a flag. He has his Sherpa take a picture of him on that peak with his flag. And then he gets his ass down off that peak so he can breathe without an oxygen canister.

If he's a serious climber, he probably goes out the next year and climbs a higher peak. Or, if there isn't a higher one, he finds one that's challenging in a different way—maybe it's inhabited by a yeti. And when he reaches the top, he races back down off that one, too.

Compare that mountaineer to a guy like you: You launched a weightlifting and diet program—the one in this book, say. You achieved terrific results—maybe you lost 15 pounds and got notably stronger. You can look in the mirror and see all kinds of stuff you didn't see before:

What was once as smooth as paste is now an emerging topographical map of muscles and veins. What once flowed over your belt like volcanic sludge is now flat and almost solid.

This is terrific—a marked difference. But it's not the promised land. It's not Nirvana. It's not the body on the cover of *Men's Health*. So instead of recognizing that you're standing on a nice little peak, you decide you're just at a higher level of base camp, and now you're going to begin the *real* climb.

Bad idea. You should follow the example of that climber: When he reaches the top of a mountain, he doesn't immediately run over to the first mountain on the left and start climbing that one. (For one thing, there's usually a nice little abyss in between.) He acknowledges that he bagged a peak and leaves the next one for another time, another expedition.

This analogy isn't perfect, of course. There's no way you want to work off 20 pounds of fat and pack on a few pounds of muscle only to go back down to where you started. So the real question is, how do you get from one peak to the next without ending up on a plateau?

Here's your plan.

1. GIVE YOUR BODY A BREAK

Now that you've reached the end of the 9-week Testosterone Advantage Workout, you're probably stronger than you've ever been. Even if you're not beating the best-ever bench press of your fabled youth, you're almost certainly using more weight on other exercises, such as lat pulldowns, squats, rows.

So it's time to back off and give your body a chance to recover. Progress comes at a price. Your muscles and connective tissues have been under increasing stress. Keep that stress up, and something will give out. Give your body a 1-week break, and it figures out how to repair itself.

This week doesn't have to be spent on the couch—you probably couldn't spend a week lying around even if you wanted to, because with a new body comes new energy. If you're anything like the guys in our pilot program, you're finding that it's become hard work to just sit and do nothing.

So play a couple of rounds of golf, go to the batting cage and hit some balls, swim, hike, ride. You can even toss around some light weights. Just don't follow a formal program, and don't lift really heavy weights.

2. PICK A NEW GOAL

One reason you were so successful in the Testosterone Advantage Plan is that you started with a goal. Whatever it was—bulking up, losing blubber, changing your body composition—you built your diet around that goal and then hit the gym with that end in sight in every workout.

Now it's time to find a new goal. Do you want to lose more fat or gain more muscle? Did you find the heavy weights in phase 3 of the workout program so much to your liking that you want to get even stronger? Do you wonder how a nice six-pack of abs would look on that newly flat waistline of yours? Do you want to see another half-inch on your upper arms?

Great. Just make sure you know exactly what your goal is before you launch your next program. For motivational purposes, it's important to have short-term and long-term goals. Short-term goals could be ones you set as frequently as every workout or every week. Long-term goals, such as those just mentioned, might take 1 year or longer to achieve.

3. PULL OUT THE CALENDAR

Next, you need to give yourself a specific deadline for reaching your long-term goal. Choose a natural break in your schedule: an extended holiday weekend, a summer vacation, a week-long business trip, an out-of-town wedding. If the break is 3 weeks away, you know that your new program—or at least the first phase of it—should be 3 weeks long.

Conversely, if the break is really far away—more than 12 weeks—you may want to set your sights on two goals: one that can be reached in the first half of the time frame, another that can be reached in the second. So if you have, say, 17 weeks to work with, you might decide the first 8 weeks will be an all-out muscle-building program. After a 1-week break, the next 8 could be geared toward fat burning.

Make sure these goals are reasonably attainable in your allotted time frame. If you reach one ahead of schedule, great! Celebrate, then set a new goal. If you don't reach your goals in the amount of time you've set, that's okay. You're still a whole lot closer to reaching them than you were before you started, so just reschedule them with more realistic expectations.

4. FIND A PROGRAM THAT FITS YOUR SCHEDULE

This book happens to have a 9-week program. There's nothing magical about 9 weeks. We wanted a program that would give you some sort of tangible results before 10 weeks, because, to be perfectly honest, the difference between 9 weeks and 10 weeks is like the difference between $9.99 and $10—the lower number just sounds better. Don't get us wrong. It isn't all about marketing. First and foremost, we wanted a time frame that was appropriate for the sorts of gains we hoped to deliver. After all, 5 weeks sounds even better than 9 weeks, so if marketing were our sole consideration, we would've gone with 5 weeks, if not less. But we knew we couldn't guarantee measurable improvements in that short a time.

There are plenty of resources to help you pick a program. *Men's Health* magazine has a range of workouts, from 3 weeks to 6 months in duration, available in reprint form at www.menshealth.com. And we could name off the tops of our heads dozens of other books, Web sites, magazines, and software programs that feature workouts of every conceivable length, for any conceivable goal.

If your search fails to turn up what you're looking for, you can always ask a trainer to design a program that fits your individual time frame and goals. This shouldn't cost a lot of money. The average trainer will jump at the chance to work with a guy who's motivated enough to seek him out and disciplined enough to follow through.

5. MAKE SURE THERE'S SOMETHING NEW IN THE PROGRAM

There's an old saying about life that's especially apt in the gym:

If you do what you've always done,
you'll get what you've always gotten.

This is why you see guys laboring away at weights for years without making any appreciable progress. They find a range of exercises and training techniques that they like (or worse, that are comfortable for them), and they doggedly keep at it despite the fact that their muscles made most of the adaptations they were ever going to make in the first 2 months. All the years after that, therefore, are a wash.

A new program should include something novel, some elements your body hasn't had a chance to adapt to yet. Those could include:

DIFFERENT EXERCISES. This is the easiest variable to manipulate. There are dozens of variations on the basic barbell biceps curl, and most guys haven't tried half of them. It is a little harder to find effective variations on the bench press, however, so you also need . . .

DIFFERENT WAYS OF DOING THE SAME EXERCISES. You can manipulate sets, repetitions, repetition speed, and rest intervals to get different results from a familiar exercise, such as the bench press. For example, in phase 3 of the T workout, you did five sets of five repetitions. And let's say that, before doing the T program, you traditionally did bench press sets in the standard light-to-heavy configuration: a set of 12, followed by a set of 8 to 10, followed by a set of 5 or 6, followed by a set of 3 or 4. That means your body has now adapted to two of the most effective systems of sets and repetitions.

So for something different, try a "wave" system of repetitions: 7, 5, 3, 7, 5, 3. Your goal is to use more weight on the second wave than you used on the first. For example, if the first set of 7 is with 135 pounds, you might start with 140 for the second wave.

DIFFERENT ORDER OF EXERCISES. If we had to guess, we'd say 90 percent of longtime weight lifters start each week's workouts with the bench press. These guys could make progress simply by starting their workouts with back or leg exercises. For example, if you've never done squats or deadlifts at the beginning of the week, when you're fresh and well-fed, you've probably never done them with full intensity. You can pack on a lot of muscle in a hurry by giving your lower body the attention you normally lavish on your chest and biceps.

DIFFERENT TRAINING SPLITS. Another rut most lifters fall into is working the same muscle groups together (called a training split) for years on end. Let's say your favorite split works your chest, shoulders, and triceps together on Monday; your back and biceps on Wednesday; and your legs on Friday. Deciding to work your quadriceps and biceps on Monday; your chest, back, and shoulders on Wednesday; and your hamstrings and triceps on Friday puts new emphasis on formerly neglected muscles and leads to noticeable improvements.

Another manipulation few long-term lifters are willing to try is a shift back to total-body workouts. Most guys eventually end up with a training split that works each muscle group once a week, twice at most. So a temporary shift back to total-body workouts—one exercise for each muscle group, three times a week—can produce surprising results. Your individual muscles have to adapt to doing three workouts a week instead of one, and the shock of the transition leads to new development.

DIFFERENT VOLUME. Phase 3 of the basic T program included three workouts of 17 sets each. That may be more or less volume than you were accustomed to (it's certainly more if you didn't work out at all before launching into the T program). But it's by no means the only possible volume. You can increase that for a few weeks, going up to, say, 24 sets in a workout. (Many trainers today believe that 24 is the upper limit for any workout; beyond that, you're probably putting yourself at risk of overtraining.) Or you can go down as low as 8 sets—say, 1 set each of eight exercises for as many muscle groups.

If you go to either extreme, make sure it's for a short duration (we recommend 3 weeks or six workouts, whichever comes first). You should make terrific adaptations at first, but diminishing returns will set in quickly.

DIFFERENT INTENSITY. This one seemed so obvious we almost left it out, but some guys still don't understand it. You probably have figured out by now that heavier weights are the key to strength and muscle gains. But you shouldn't always lift the heaviest weights possible. For one thing, you invite injury if your workouts are all heavy, all the time. For another, your body stops making progress if you never change things around (as if you hadn't heard this a dozen times already in this chapter alone). Finally, you get bored if you do the same old thing month after month and year after year.

This is why the world's top athletes use what's called periodized training (see page 292). They start preseason workouts with some type of break-in program (usually high-repetition sets with relatively light weights), then shift to hypertrophy workouts (sets of 8 to 12 repetitions of the best muscle-building exercises), and then, closer to the start of the season, move to pure-strength workouts. When the season begins, they shift to strength- and muscle-maintenance workouts.

Even if you're not an athlete, it's still a good idea to train like one. That is, spend different parts of your "season" developing pure muscle and pure strength, and work in regular breaks for your body and mind.

6. CHOOSE A DIET THAT MATCHES YOUR GOAL

You saw in the 9-week T program how coordinated diet and exercise programs work in tandem to produce greater results than you'd get from either by itself. So now you have to figure out what you need to eat to achieve your next goal. First, go back to chapter 9 and recalculate your protein and calorie needs. You may need to adjust the metabolic part of the equation. For example, if you chose "inactive" for the 9-week T program, you may want to change that to "moderately active" or even "very active" for your next program. That means that, to achieve the same results, you'll eat more calories along with a lower percentage of calories from protein and greater percentages from fat and carbohydrate.

A second consideration is your dietary goal. If you decide you want to go for a defined six-pack, you probably have to choose a fat-loss diet to pull it off. You'll get your six-pack sooner if you set out to take off 5 pounds of fat in 5 weeks than if you try to maintain your weight while

Periodized Training

An NBA player who's just finished a 6-month season probably takes a month off, doing nothing more than playing golf and servicing any women he was too tired to entertain during the season.

Then he starts his preseason workouts with some type of break-in program—probably featuring high-repetition sets with relatively light weights. This prepares his muscles, joints, and connective tissues for the more serious conditioning work to come.

The next stage of his training is probably focused on hypertrophy, which features sets of 8 to 12 repetitions of the best muscle-building exercises. Closer to the start of preseason practices, he segues to pure strength-building workouts.

Once practices start, he scales back on lifting and focuses on sport-specific drills, allowing his bigger, stronger muscles to relearn hoops basics.

Then comes the regular season, when his body takes tremendous pounding, day in and day out. He needs to maintain his strength, or he won't make it through in one piece. But if he overdoes it in the weight room, he puts too much stress on his body and causes it to break down even faster.

Once his season ends, he takes a month off, and does it all over again. Welcome to the wonderful world of periodized training.

How do you put this to work for you? Let's say your "season" is the summer, when you spend weekends at the community pool. When you aren't at the pool, you do some heavy yard work. All this cuts into your workout time, on top of the double-whammy of putting stress on your body in the yard and putting your body on display at the pool.

So you begin to prepare in January. You start with high-repetition workouts, then shift to some serious muscle-building routines in February. In March, you focus more on building strength—setting new personal records in the squat and bench press, perhaps. In April, you shift to the vanity muscles, trying to put some new meat on your arms and shoulders. Then in May, you attack body fat and work on your abs.

By pool season, you're bigger and leaner than you were at the same time the year before. For the next 3 months, you do light workouts a couple of times a week, keeping the fat in check and the muscles looking sharp. Your goal is just to hold on to your physique until the pool closes, your boss returns from vacation, and you have to start working those 12-hour days again.

building new muscle, because it's faster to take off fat than to put on muscle.

7. START SLOWLY

Want to make sure a new workout program fails? Start the first week of workouts by using the heaviest weights you can lift. Even if you're in the best shape of your life, you still need to give your body a chance to get used to the new elements of your exercises, your new workout schedule, your new system of sets and repetitions—all the stuff we discussed above in more detail than you probably cared to know.

Ideally, the first week of a new program should be a break-in phase, in which you use weights you're sure you can handle on all exercises. In the second week, you can start pushing yourself and using the heaviest weights possible for whatever system of sets and repetitions you've chosen. Then, in the third week, you can graduate to heavier weights than you've ever used before.

8. WHEN YOU REACH THE PEAK, TAKE YOUR SNAPSHOT—THEN GET THE HELL OFF

In fitness and in life, many plateaus are self-imposed: You convince yourself that you've gone as far as you can go. We urge you to keep challenging yourself (within the sensible limits we've described above and elsewhere in this book, of course). With new goals every few weeks, you'll never get bored; rarely, if ever, get hurt; and always have a reason to look forward to the next workout. Take it from us: That's one of the best feelings a guy can have.

So when you get your six-pack or your 225-pound bench press or your 34-inch waist, celebrate, tell your friends, download pictures of yourself onto your personal Web page—and then repeat these 8 steps all over again.

Forever.

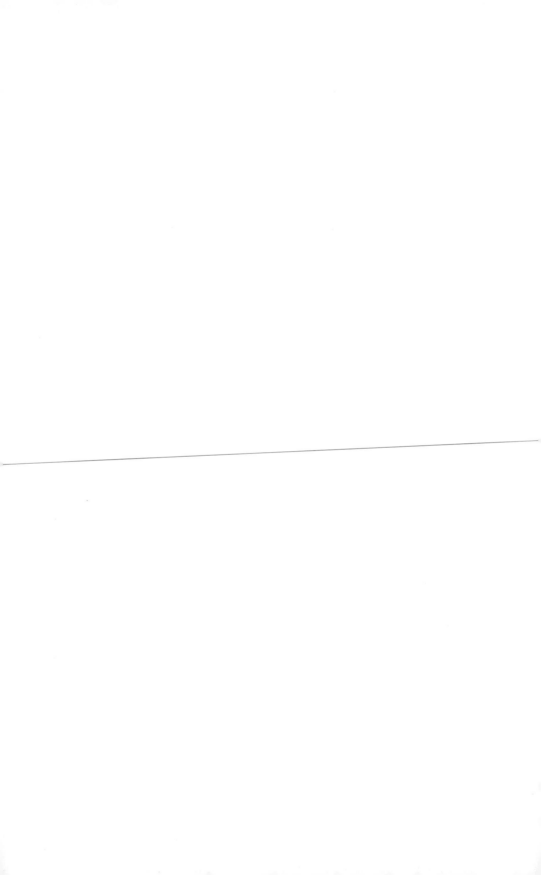

ABOUT THE AUTHORS

Lou Schuler, fitness director of *Men's Health* magazine, has written on male fitness and strength training for over a decade. He is certified by the National Strength and Conditioning Association as a certified-strength-and-conditioning-specialist (C.S.C.S.), the top credential in the field of personal training. Schuler and his wife, Kimberly Heinrichs, live with their three children in Allentown, Pennsylvania.

Jeff Volek, R.D., Ph.D., C.S.C.S., a professor attached to the acclaimed Human Performance Laboratory at the University of Connecticut, has published often on fitness and athletic performance. While at Ball State University in Indiana, Dr. Volek was among the first researchers to uncover and study the link between diet and testosterone. He lives in Manchester, Connecticut.

Michael Mejia, C.S.C.S., has been a personal trainer in New York City since 1993, working with a clientele that ranges from elite athletes to corporate CEOs. He writes often on fitness and is a contributing editor and exercise advisor to *Men's Health*. Mejia and his wife, Michelle, live with their two children in Plainview, Long Island.

Adam Campbell, C.S.C.S., is assistant fitness editor at *Men's Health*. He worked in clinical weight loss for 2 years and specializes in translating body-composition goals into specific food plans. Campbell and his wife, Stefanie, live in Trexlertown, Pennsylvania.

INDEX

Underscored page references indicate boxed text. **Boldface** references indicate photographs or illustrations.

A

Abdominal muscles, <u>194</u>, **194**
  stretch for, 189, **189**
Actin, 64
Activity level, 95
ADD, <u>8</u>
Adrenaline, 34, 49, 164
Aerobic exercise, 31–36
  cortisol increase from, 164, 165
  examples of, 33
  metabolic effects of, 39, 40
  muscle adaptation to, 36
  problems with, 4–5, 31–33
    heart-rhythm disturbances, 32
    injuries, 32
    joint pain, 9, 43
    muscle decrease, 9, 32, 34, 39
    tendinitis, 43
    testosterone decrease, 40
  strength training combined with, 41

Aerobic fitness
  improving with weight loss, 36
  VO_2 max as measure of, 35–36
Aerobics movement, history of, 36–39
Age, muscle mass and, <u>159</u>
Alcohol, effects of, <u>62–63</u>
Alzheimer's disease, 52–53, 69
Amino acids, 75, 93
Anabolic steroids, 45, 109
Anabolism, 74
Anatomical adaptation, 166
AndroGel, 49–50, 53
Androstenediol supplements, <u>174, 176</u>
Androstenedione supplements, <u>174–76</u>
Angina, 22
Antibodies, 64
Antioxidants, in chocolate, 140
Appetite, <u>7–8</u>
Arm length, <u>158–59</u>

Assisted pullup, 271, **271**
Asthma, obesity as cause of, 23–24
Attention deficit disorder (ADD), 8

B

Back, stretches for
 lower, 186, **186**
 upper, 183, **183**
Back extension, **220**, 221, **251**
Barbell bench press, 233, **233**,
  263, **263**
Barbell concentration curl, 241,
  241, 281, **281**
Barbells, 171, **171**
Barbell shoulder press, 238, **238**
Basal metabolism. *See* Metabolism,
  basal
Before & After, 12, 14
 Hoye, Mike, 81
 Kelleher, J. C., 37
 Kemler, Greg, 51
 Schmaldinst, Cory, 15
 Smith, Mike, 111
 Stash, Ed, 25
Bench press
 barbell, 233, **233**, 263, **263**
 injuries from, 168
 spotter for, 190
Biceps, 191, **191**
Biceps curl, seated dumbbell, 219,
  219
Biceps femoris, 195, **195**
Bladder cancer, 72
Blindness, diabetes and, 23
Blood pressure
 high
  health consequences of, 22
  incidence of, 22
  from Meridia, 103
  obesity and, 22
  polymetabolic syndrome and,
   163

 measurements, 22
 sleep apnea and, 27
Blood sugar, 90, 108
Bone density, 24
Bone loss, 69–70
Bounce, avoiding, during lifting, 199
Brachialis, 191, **191**
Brachioradialis, 191
Brain chemistry, obesity and, 8
Breads, glycemic index of, 92
Breakfast
 benefits of, 107–8
 menus, for
  cruiserweight, 133–39
  heavyweight, 119–25
  welterweight, 145–51
Break-in program, 291, 292
Butter, 85

C

Cable row, 234, **234**
Caffeine, 152
Calcium, 69–70
Calf muscles, 195, **195**
 stretch for, 188, **188**
Calf raise
 free-weight seated, 253, **253**
 one-legged standing, 274, **274**
 seated, 252, **252**
 standing, 215, **215**
Calories
 burning, 17
 daily consumption of, 7
 in
  supplements, 110, 112
  Testosterone Advantage Plan
   diet, 95, 96, 97
Cancer
 bladder, 72
 incidence factors
  fitness level, 22–23
  free radicals, 44

genetics, 23
obesity, 23
prostate, 87, 89
Canola oil, 84
Carbohydrate, 88–93
calories per gram of, 99
classification of, 89
complex, 89, 92
consumption of, recommended
by
Food Guide Pyramid, 10
low-carbohydrate diets, 101–2
postexercise meal, 93, 108–9
Testosterone Advantage Plan
diet, **57–59**, 58–60
glycemic index of, 90–93
simple, 89, 92
thermic effect of feeding and, 67
Cardiovascular disease. *See* Heart
disease
Catabolism, 74–75
Cereals, glycemic index of, 91
Chemical bonds, energy in, 66
Chest press, machine, 206, **206**
Chest stretch, 183, **183**
Chinese food, 129
Chinup bar, 170, **170**
Chocolate, antioxidants in, 140
Cholesterol, 79–80, 82–86
obesity and, 22
testosterone and, 46
Circuits in phase-1 workout, 199
Coffee, 152
Cola, 152
Compliance, with
diet, 66, 89, 102
fitness regimens, 29
Food Guide Pyramid
recommendations, 10
Compound set, 191
Concentration curl, barbell, 241,
241, 281, **281**

Condiments, choosing, 127
Copper, 177
Cornstarch, 93
Corn syrup, high-fructose, 7
Coronary arteries, 50, 52
Cortisol, 63, 163–64, 177
Cost, of workout equipment vs. gym
membership, 167–68
Creatine, 174
Cruiserweight
grocery list, 132
menus, 133–39
protein shake, 115
Crunch, 218, **218**
dumbbell reverse, 283, **283**
incline reverse, 282, **282**
reverse, 254, **254**
Swiss-ball, 243, **243**
with towel, 244, **244**
Curl
barbell concentration, 241, **241**,
281, **281**
dumbbell leg, 209, **209**, 249
preacher, 240, **240**, 280,
280
seated dumbbell biceps, 219,
219
seated leg, 265, **265**

D

Dairy products, 91, 101
Deadlift, 262, **262**
Decline pushup, 207
Deltoids, **191**, 192
Dexfenfluramine, 103
Diabetes, 23, 44
Diet(s)
compliance to, 66, 89, 102
goals
bulk up, 58, **58**
lose fat, **57**, 58
maintain weight, 59, **59**

Diet(s) (*cont.*)
    guidelines from U. S.
        government, 9
    meal-replacement supplements
        and, 109–10, 112
    postexercise meal, 108–9
    pre-exercise meal, 112–13
    types of
        higher-fat, 19, 86–87
        high-protein, 69–70, <u>73</u>
        high-sugar, <u>7–8</u>
        low-carbohydrate, 101–2
        low-fat, 9, 18, 102
        Mediterranean, 87, 102
        Testosterone Advantage Plan
            (*see* Testosterone Advantage
            Plan diet)
        vegetarian, 76, 86
Dietary sugar. *See also*
        Carbohydrate
    calories per teaspoon of, <u>7</u>
    glycemic index of, 92
    simple, 89
Diet pills, <u>103</u>
Dinner menus, for
    cruiserweight, 133–39
    heavyweight, 119–25
    welterweight, 145–51
Dinner recipes. *See* Recipes
Diuretics, cola and coffee as,
    <u>152</u>
Dopamine, obesity and, <u>8</u>
Dumbbell external rotation, 242,
    242
Dumbbell leg curl, 209, **209**, **249**
Dumbbell leg extension, 213, **213**,
    250
Dumbbell reverse crunch, 283, **283**
Dumbbell row, one-arm, 211, **211**
Dumbbells, 172, **172**
Dumbbell stepup, 272, **272**

E

Endurance exercise. *See* Aerobic
    exercise
Energy
    balance, 100–101
    from chemical bonds, 66
Enzymes, 64
Epinephrine, 164
Equipment, for home workout,
    170–72
    barbell, 170, **171**
    chinup bar, 170, **170**
    dumbbells, **171**, 172
    EZ-curl bar, 170, **171**
    weight bench, 170, **170**
    weight plates, **171**, 171–72
Erectile problems, low testosterone
    and, 49
Erector spinae, **193**, <u>193</u>
Essential amino acids, 75
Essential fatty acids, 84
Estrogen
    Alzheimer's disease and,
        53
    gynecomastia from, <u>176</u>
    osteoporosis and, 24
    prohormone supplementation
        and, <u>176</u>
Exercise(s). *See also* Aerobic
        exercise; Weight lifting
    duration of, 28–30
    fuels for, 33–34
    gym
        back extension, **220**, 221, **251**
        barbell bench press, 233, **233**,
            263, **263**
        barbell shoulder press, 238,
            238
        cable row, 234, **234**
        crunch, 218, **218**
        deadlift, 262, **262**
        dumbbell external rotation,

242, **242**
dumbbell stepup, 272, **272**
lateral raise, 214, **214**
lat pulldown, 236, **236**
leg curl, 208, **208**, 249
leg extension, 212, **212**, **250**
leg press, 204, **204**, **248**
lying triceps extension with EZ
    bar, 239, **239**
machine chest press, 206, **206**
machine row, 216, **216**
military press, 279, **279**
one-arm row (elbow out), 264,
    264
one-legged standing calf raise,
    274, **274**
overhead triceps extension,
    273, **273**
preacher curl, 240, **240**, 280,
    280
reverse crunch, 254, **254**
seated calf raise, 252, **252**
seated leg curl, 265, **265**
squat, 278, **278**
Swiss-ball crunch, 243, **243**
triceps pushdown, 222, **222**
underhand-grip lat pulldown,
    210, **210**
wide-grip lat pulldown, 270,
    270
home
    assisted pullup, 271, **271**
    barbell bench press, 233, **233**,
        263, **263**
    barbell concentration curl,
        241, **241**, 281, **281**
    barbell shoulder press, 239,
        239
    crunch with towel, 244, **244**
    deadlift, 262, **262**
    dumbbell external rotation,
        242, **242**

dumbbell leg curl, 209, **209**,
    248
dumbbell leg extension, 213,
    213, **250**
dumbbell stepup, 272, **272**
free-weight seated calf raise,
    253, **253**
hip extension, 266, **266**
lying dumbbell triceps
    extension, 223, **223**
lying triceps extension with EZ
    bar, 239, **239**
military press, 279, **279**
one-arm dumbbell row, 211,
    211, 235, **235**
one-arm row (elbow out), 264,
    264
one-legged standing calf raise,
    274, **274**
overhead triceps extension,
    273, **273**
pushup, 207, **207**
reverse crunch, 254, **254**
reverse fly, 217, **217**
reverse pushup, 237, **237**
seated dumbbell biceps curl,
    219, **219**
split squat, 205, **205**, **248**
squat, 278, **278**
standing calf raise, 215, **215**
superman, 221, **221**, **251**
after meals, 108–9
osteoporosis prevented with,
    24
physiology, 33–34
recovery from, 108
weight loss and, 155–56
variations, 289–91
External obliques, **194**, <u>194</u>
EZ-curl bar, 170, **171**

F

Fast food, _126–28_
Fast-twitch muscle fibers, _158_,
_160_
Fat, dietary, 77–80, 82–87
  alcohol and, _62–63_
  calories per gram of, 99
  essential fatty acids, 84
  as fuel for exercise, 33–34
  in Mediterranean diet, 87
  recommendations for
      consumption of, 12
    Food Guide Pyramid, 10–11
    Testosterone Advantage Plan,
      57–59, 58–60
  testosterone and, 12, 86–87
  thermic effect of feeding and,
      67, 77
  types of
    monounsaturated, 84, 85,
      87
    omega-3 fatty acids, 84, 85
    omega-6 fatty acids, 84, 85
    partially hydrogenated, 85
    polyunsaturated, 84
    saturated, 83, 84, 85
    trans, 84–85
Fat-soluble vitamins, 12
Fatty acids, 10, 84, 85
Feeding, thermic effect of, 17,
    18
Fenfluramine, _103_
Fen-phen, _103_
Fish, as source of
  linolenic acid, 84
  omega-3 fatty acids, 10, 84
  polyunsaturated fats, 84
Fitness, 21–30
  as abstraction, 28
  for improvements in
    functional limitations, 26
    health, 21–24

income, 27
sex, 27
sleep, 27
Fixx, Jim, 31, 38
Flaxseed oil, 84
Flexibility, 42
  sports performance and, 180
  warmups and, 173
  weight lifting and, 180
Fluid
  intake
    benefits of increased, _72_
    requirements, _73_
    in Testosterone Advantage
      Plan, _72–73_
  loss
    calculating, _73_
    sources of, 69, _72_, _73_
Fly
  reverse, 217, **217**
Food Guide Pyramid, **9**
  compliance with, 11
  creation of, 9
  errors and inconsistencies in,
      10–11
  failure of, 4
  heart disease and, 11
  protein recommendations, 58
Free radicals, 44
Free-weight seated calf raise, 253,
    253
French press, 273
Fructose, 89
Fruits, 10, 91

G

Gallbladder disease, 24
Gastrointestinal distress, from
      protein bars, 112
Genetics, influence of, on
  arm length, _158–59_
  cancer, 23

cholesterol metabolism and
  absorption, 82
fat storage, 8
muscle fiber, 158
muscle length, 159
perspiration, 73
tendon attachment point,
  159
VO₂ max, 35
GH, 162–63
GI, 91–92
Giant set, 191
Glucose, 7–8, 90
Glucose tolerance, weight training
  and, 44
Gluteus muscles, 193, **195**
  stretch for, 186, **186**
Glycemic index (GI), 91–92
Glycerol in protein bars, 112
Glycogen
  aerobic training and, 41
  depleted by exercise, 92–93
  fluid loss and, 69
  as fuel for exercise, 33–34
Goals
  matching
    diet and exercise, 291
    workout program to, 288
  setting new, 287–88
  Testosterone Advantage Plan diet
    calculations and, 96–97
Gout, 24
Grains, 10, 91
Grocery list
  cruiserweight, 132
  heavyweight, 118
  welterweight, 144
Growth hormone (GH), 162–63
Guacamole, fat in, 129
Gym
  equipment (see Equipment, for
    home workout)

exercises (see Exercise(s),
    gym)
  location considerations, 167–69
Gynecomastia, 176

H

Hamstring muscles, 195, **195**
  stretch for, 187, **187**
HDL. See High-density lipoprotein
Health benefits of fitness and fat
    loss, 21–24
Heart disease
  aerobic exercise and, 32
  causes of
    diabetes, 23
    diet pills, 103
    free radicals, 44
    genetics, 38
    high blood pressure, 22
    obesity, 22
  cholesterol and, 79–80, 82–83
  decreasing risk of, with
    higher-fat diet, 86
    physical activity, 30
  Food Guide Pyramid and, 11
  increased risk of, from
    alcohol, 63
    high-protein diet, 70
  in polymetabolic syndrome,
    163
  preventing, with
    sexual activity, 54
    strength training, 43, 44
    testosterone, 50, 52
  sleep apnea and, 27
  triglycerides and, 80, 82
Heavyweight
  grocery list, 118
  menus, 119–25
  protein shake, 115
Hemoglobin, 64
Herbal supplements, 176–77

High-density lipoprotein (HDL), 80, 82–85
  benefits of, 80
  elevating, with
    dietary fat, 83–84
    monounsaturated fats, 84, 85
  lowered by trans fats, 85
Hip, stretch for, 186, **186**
Hip extension, 266, **266**
Hip flexors, 181, **194**, <u>194–95</u>
  stretch for, 188, **188**
Home exercises. *See* Exercise(s), home
Hormones. *See specific hormones*
Hoye, Mike, <u>81</u>
Hunger. *See also* Satiety
  food cravings, 101
  high-glycemic meal and, 90
Hydration, <u>72–73</u>
Hydrogenation, 85
Hygiene, at gym, 168
Hypertrophy, 167, 226

I

Iliacus, **194**, <u>194</u>
Immune system, testosterone and, 46
Impotence, diabetes as cause of, 23
Incline reverse crunch, 282, **282**
Income, fitness and, 27
Infraspinatus, **191**, <u>192</u>
Insulin, 163
  appetite and, <u>7–8</u>
  glucose and, 90
  high-sugar diet and, <u>7–8</u>
  to prevent protein breakdown, 93, 109
  to promote protein synthesis, 93, 109
  release signal, 90, 93, 108–9
  resistance, 90, 163
  syndrome X and, 163

Intensity, of workout, 290–91
Internal obliques, **194**, <u>194</u>
Internal rotator cuff, stretch for, 185, **185**

J

Joint disease/pain
  aerobic exercise and, 9, 32, 43
  gout, 24
  osteoarthritis, 24
  runner's knee, 32
Juice. *See* Testosterone

K

Kelleher, J. C., <u>37</u>
Kemler, Greg, <u>51</u>
Kidney disease
  causes of
    diabetes, 23
    high-protein diet, 69
  fluid intake to prevent, <u>72</u>
  kidney stones, <u>72</u>

L

Lactate threshold, 34
Lactic acid, growth hormone and, 163
Lactose, 89, 112
Lateral raise, 214, **214**
Latissimus dorsi, <u>192–93</u>, **193**
Lat pulldown, 236, **236**
  underhand-grip, 210, **210**
  wide-grip, 270, **270**
LDL. *See* Low-density lipoprotein
Leg curl, **249**
  dumbbell, 209, **209**, **249**
  seated, 208, **208**, 265, **265**
Leg extension, 212, **212**, **250**
  dumbbell, 213, **213**, **250**
Leg press, 204, **204**, **248**
Legumes, glycemic index of, 91
Leptin, appetite and, <u>7–8</u>

Libido, testosterone and, 49
Linoleic acid, 84
Linolenic acid, 84
Liver disease, 63
Log, workout. *See* Workout log
Low-density lipoprotein (LDL), 80,
    82–85
  dangers from, 80
  increased by
    saturated fat, 83, 85
    trans fats, 85
Lunch menus, for
  cruiserweight, 133–39
  heavyweight, 119–25
  welterweight, 145–51
Luteninizing hormone, 176
Lying dumbbell triceps extension,
    223, **223**
Lying triceps extension with EZ bar,
    239, **239**

M

Macadamia nuts, 84
Machine chest press, 206, **206**
Machine row, 216, **216**
Macronutrient balance, 101
Macronutrients. *See* Carbohydrate;
    Fat; Protein
Magnesium supplementation,
    177
Maltodextrin, 93
Marathoner, fitness of, 16
Margarine, 85
Mayonnaise, 127
McGwire, Mark, 175, 176
Meal planner, 114
  cruiserweight, 132–39
  heavyweight, 118–25
  welterweight, 144–51
Meals. *See also* Menus
  breakfast, 107–8
  number of, 105–7
  postexercise, 108–9
  pre-exercise, 112–13
Meal supplements, 109–10, 112
Mediterranean diet, 87, 102
Men's Health T, 12, 57–60, **57, 58,**
    59
Menus
  cruiserweight, 133–39
  heavyweight, 119–25
  in pilot program, 13
  welterweight, 145–51
Meridia, 103
Metabolic weight, 41, 67, 157
Metabolism
  basal, 17, 39, 40
  Testosterone Advantage Plan and,
    94–96
Mexican food, 129
Military press, 279, **279**
Milk, 91, 101
Mixed grip, 262
Monounsaturated fats, 84, 87
Multijoint exercise, 234
Multiplier effect, 104
Muscle(s)
  aerobic exercise and, 36
  age and, 34, 159
  anabolism of, 74
  catabolism of, 74–75
  damage from weight lifting, 74
  decrease from
    aerobic exercise, 9, 32, 34, 39
    age, 34
    alcohol, 62, 63
    vegetarian diet, 76
  energy requirements of, 26
  fiber types, 34, 158, 160
    conversion of, from fast-
      twitch to slow-twitch,
      160–61
  gain, rate of, 98
  hypertrophy, 226

Muscle(s) (*cont.*)
  increasing, with
    meat, 76
    stretching, 181
    testosterone supplementation,
      47–48
  lactic-acid buildup in, 34
  length, <u>159</u>
  metabolism and, 17, 40
  structure, 64
  types of
    abdominals, <u>194</u>, **194**
    biceps, <u>191</u>, **191**
    biceps femoris, <u>195</u>, **195**
    brachialis, <u>191</u>, **191**
    brachioradialis, <u>191</u>
    calf, <u>195</u>, **195**
    deltoids, **191**, <u>192</u>
    erector spinae, <u>193</u>, **193**
    external obliques, <u>194</u>, **194**
    gastrocnemius, <u>195</u>, **195**
    gluteals, <u>193</u>, **195**
    hamstrings, <u>195</u>, **195**
    hip flexors, **194**, <u>194–95</u>
    iliacus, <u>194</u>, **194**
    infraspinatus, **191**, <u>192</u>
    internal obliques, <u>194</u>, **194**
    latissimus dorsi, <u>192–93</u>, **193**
    pectorals, <u>194</u>, **194**
    psoas major, <u>194</u>, **194**
    psoas minor, <u>194</u>, **194**
    quadriceps, <u>195</u>, **195**
    rectus abdominis, <u>194</u>, **194**
    rectus femoris, <u>195</u>, **195**
    rotator cuff, <u>192</u>
    semimembranosus, <u>195</u>, **195**
    semitendinosus, <u>195</u>, **195**
    soleus, <u>195</u>, **195**
    spinal erectors, <u>193</u>, **193**
    subscapularis, **191**, <u>192</u>
    supraspinatus, **191**, <u>192</u>
    teres minor, **191**, <u>192</u>
    transverse abdominis, <u>194</u>, **194**
    trapezius, <u>192</u>, **193**
    triceps, <u>192</u>, **193**
    vastus intermedius, <u>195</u>, **195**
    vastus lateralis, <u>195</u>, **195**
    vastus medialis, <u>195</u>, **195**
  warmup procedure for, 172–73,
    178–79
Myoplex, 69
Myosin, 64

N

Neck, stretch for, 184, **184**
Neurological function, testosterone
  and, 46
Nitrogen balance, 64–65
Norandrodiol, <u>176</u>
Nortestosterone, <u>176</u>
Nutritional supplements, <u>174–77</u>
  ZMA, <u>177</u>
Nuts, 84

O

Obesity
  cereal and, 107
  health risks associated with
    asthma, 23–24
    cancer, 22–23
    death, 20–21
    diabetes, 23
    gallbladder disease, 24
    gout, 24
    heart disease, 22
    high blood pressure, 22
    osteoarthritis, 24
    osteoporosis, 24
    sleep apnea, 27
    stroke, 22
  incidence of, 4, <u>6</u>
Obliques, <u>194</u>, **194**
Olive oil, 84, 87
Olympic bar, 171, **171**

Omega-3 fatty acids, 10, 84, 85
Omega-6 fatty acids, 84, 85
One-arm dumbbell row, 211, **211**, 235, **235**
One-arm row (elbow out), 264, **264**
One-legged standing calf raise, 274, **274**
One-rep max (1RM), <u>190</u>
Osteoarthritis, 24
Osteoporosis, 24
Overeating, reasons for, <u>7–8</u>
Overhead triceps extension, 273, **273**
Overweight. *See* Obesity
Oxygen utilization, testosterone and, 46

P

Pasta, 91, <u>126</u>
Pastries, glycemic index of, 92
Pectorals, <u>194</u>, **194**
Peptide hormone, 162–63
Periodized training, <u>292</u>
Phosphorus, 70
Pilot program for Testosterone Advantage Plan, <u>13–14</u>, 19, 60, <u>98</u>, 102
Piriformis, 181
Pizza, <u>128</u>
Plateau, 285–86, 293
Polymetabolic syndrome, 163
Polyunsaturated fats, 84
Postexercise
  meals, 108–9
  supplements, 109–10, 112
Preacher curl, 240, **240**, 280, **280**
Pre-exercise meal, 112–13
Prohormones, <u>174–76</u>
Prostate cancer, 87, 89
Protein, 61, 64–71, 74–76
  animal vs. vegetable, 10
  calories per gram of, 99

effects of dietary intake of
  decreased sex-hormone-binding globulin level, 71
  fluid loss, 69, <u>73</u>
  metabolic weight control, 67
  nitrogen balance, 64
  satiety, 65
  thermic, 17–18, 66–67
essential amino acids, 75
forms of, 61, 64
health risks purportedly related to, 69–70
insulin and, 93
intake recommendations of
  Food Guide Pyramid, 10, 58
  Testosterone Advantage Plan, 58–59, 68, 76
in postexercise meal, 108–9
Protein bars, 109–10, 112
Protein shake, 109, 110, 112, 115
Psoas major, <u>194</u>, **194**
Psoas minor, <u>194</u>, **194**
Pullup
  assisted, 271, **271**
  spotter for, <u>190</u>
Pushup, 207, **207**
  decline, 207
  decline three-point, 207
  reverse, 237, **237**
  three-point, 207

Q

Quadriceps muscles, **195**, <u>195</u>
  stretch for, 188, **188**

R

Recipes
  Broiled Shrimp Scampi
    cruiserweight, 139
    heavyweight, 125
    welterweight, 151

Recipes (*cont.*)
  Chicken-and-Vegetable Stir-Fry
    cruiserweight, 133
    heavyweight, 119
    welterweight, 145
  Chili
    cruiserweight, 137
    heavyweight, 123
    welterweight, 149
  Grilled Steak
    cruiserweight, 135
    heavyweight, 121
    welterweight, 147
  Hamburgers
    cruiserweight, 138
    heavyweight, 124
    welterweight, 150
  Penne with Italian Sausage
    cruiserweight, 134
    heavyweight, 120
    welterweight, 146
  Roasted Salmon with Goat Cheese
    cruiserweight, 136
    heavyweight, 122
    welterweight, 148
Rectus abdominis, 194, **194**
Rectus femoris, 195, **195**
Redux, 103
Repetitions, 190, 199, 227, 257
Reverse crunch, 254, **254**
  dumbbell, 283, **283**
  incline, 282, **282**
Reverse fly, 217, **217**
Reverse pushup, 237, **237**
Rotator cuff, 242
  injury, 192
  muscles of, **191**, 192
  stretch for, 185, **185**
Row
  cable, 234, **234**
  machine, 216, **216**
  one-arm (elbow out), 264, **264**

one-arm dumbbell, 211, **211**, 235, **235**

S

Safflower oil, 84
Salt, 101
Satiety, from
  fat intake, 60
  high-glycemic foods, 90
  protein intake, 65
Saturated fats
  HDL elevation from, 84, 85
  LDL elevation from, 83, 84, 85
  in Mediterranean diet, 87
Schmaldinst, Cory, 15
Seated calf raise, 252, **252**
Seated dumbbell biceps curl, 219, **219**
Seated leg curl, 265, **265**
Semimembranosus, **195**, 195
Semitendinosus, **195**, 195
Serotonin, in starch-based meal, 126
Servings, waiting between, 141
Set, definition of, 190
Sex-hormone-binding globulin, 71
Sexual function, testosterone and, 49–50, 53–54
Shakes, protein, 109, 110, 112, 115
Shoulder, stretch for rear, 184, **184**
Shoulder press
  barbell, 238, **238**
Shrugs, 192
Sibutramine, 103
Side torso, stretch for, 189, **189**
Skin-fold measurements, 47
Sleep apnea, 27
Slow-twitch muscle fibers, 158
Smith, Mike, 111
Smith machine, 233, 263

Snack(s)
  glycemic index of, 91–92
  menus for
    cruiserweight, 133–39
    heavyweight, 119–25
    welterweight, 145–51
Soups, glycemic index of, 91
Sour cream, 129
Spinal erectors, **193**, 193
Split squat, 205, **205**, **248**
Spot, 190
Sprinter, fitness of, 16
Squat, 278, **278**
  range of motion and, 181
  split, 205, **205**, **248**
Standing calf raise, 215, **215**
  one-legged, 274, **274**
Stash, Ed, 25
Stepup, dumbbell, 272, **272**
Steroids, anabolic, 45, 109
Strength
  decreases in function limitations
      and, 26
  phase of workout program, 167
Strength training. *See also* Weight
      lifting
  aerobics combined with, 41
  benefits of
    blood pressure decrease, 43
    cholesterol decrease, 43
    diabetes prevention, 44
    heart health, 43–44
  flexibility and, 42
  popularity of, 39
  testosterone supplementation
      and, 47–48
  warmups for, 41
Stress hormones, 163–64
Stretch(ing)
  benefits of, 179–81
    improved sports performance,
      179–80

injury prevention, 179
muscle gain, 180–81
pain relief, 179
  duration of, 182
  for
    abdominals, 189, **189**
    calf, 188, **188**
    chest, 183, **183**
    gluteus, 186, **186**
    hamstring, 187, **187**
    hip, 186, **186**
    hip flexors, 188, **188**
    lower back, 186, **186**
    neck, 184, **184**
    quadriceps, 188, **188**
    rotator cuff, 185, **185**
    shoulder, 184, **184**
    side torso, 189, **189**
    trapezius, 184, **184**
    triceps, 185, **185**
    upper back, 183, **183**
  sequence, 182
  strength training and, 180–81
  timing of, 181–82
Stroke
  causes of, 22, 23, 44
  preventing, with sexual activity, 54
  sleep apnea and, 27
Stroke volume, improving, with
      weight training, 44
Subscapularis, 192
Sucrose, 89
Sunflower oil, 84
Superman, 221, **221**, **251**
Supersets, 191, 226–27
Supplements
  meal-replacement, 109–10, 112
  nutritional, 174–77
Supraspinatus, **191**, 192
Sweeteners, 7, 152
Sweets, 140–41
  craving for, 101

Swiss-ball crunch, 243, **243**
Syndrome X, 163
Synovial fluid, 173

T

Temperature, raising, with
warmups, 173
Tempo, workout, 199, 227, 257
Tendinitis, aerobic exercise and, 43
Tendon attachment point, 159
Teres minor, **191**, 192
Terminology, at gym, 190–95
Testosterone
benefits of, 46
Alzheimer's prevention, 52–53
cholesterol regulation, 46, 50
coronary-artery dilation, 50, 52
heart health, 50, 52
improved mood, 50
increased muscle mass, 47,
48, 161
muscle fiber conversion,
160–61
sexual, 49, 50, 53–54
strength, 47, 48
cholesterol as precursor of, 80,
86
decreased by
aerobic exercise, 40
age, 45–46
low-fat diet, 9, 18
obesity, 7, 8
protein-deficient diet, 53
sex-hormone-binding globulin,
71
vegetarian diet, 76, 86
functions of, 46
increased by
herbs, 176–77
higher-fat diet, 19, 86–87
magnesium, 177
meat, 86

prohormones, 174–76
weight training, 40, 161
zinc, 177
negative effects of, 48–49
receptors, 46, 162
secretion cycle, 45
transformation to estrogen, 24
Testosterone Advantage Plan diet
alcohol in, 62–63
breakfast in, 108
caffeine in, 152
calculations in, 94–100
carbohydrate in, 60, 89, 92, 93
in combination with Testosterone
Advantage workout, 102,
165
fast food in, 126–29
fat in, 58–59, 78, 86
saturated, 83
trans, 85
hormones and, 86
hydration in, 72–73
Kelleher, J. C., on, 37
Kemler, Greg, on, 51
meal plans for, 114–15
Mediterranean diet and, 87
Men's Health T and, 57–60
pasta in, 126
in pilot program, 60
pizza in, 128
post-workout meals in, 109
protein in, 58, 61, 68, 76
metabolism and, 66–67
protein shakes in, 115
Smith, Mike, on, 111
Stash, Ed, on, 25
sweets in, 140–42
Testosterone Advantage workout
anatomical adaptation in, 166
in combination with Testosterone
Advantage Plan diet, 102,
165

hypertrophy in, 167
phase
  1, 198–223
  2, 226–54
  3, 256–83
strength in, 167
Thermic effect of feeding, 17, 18, 66
Three-point pushup, 207
Time, as diet issue, 6
Toes, weight-lifting injuries to, 168
Torso, side, stretch for, 189, **189**
Total-body workouts, 290
Training split, 290
Trans fats, 84–85
Transporters, 64
Transverse abdominis, 194, **194**
Trapezius, stretch for, 184, **184**
Tribulus, 176–77
Triceps, 192, **193**
  stretch for, 185, **185**
Triceps extension
  lying, with EZ bar, 239, **239**
  lying dumbbell, 223, **223**
  overhead, 273, **273**
Triceps pushdown, 222, **222**
Triglycerides
  heart disease and, 79, 80, 82
  levels, 82
  lowering, 84, 85
  obesity and, 22
Triset, 191

U

Underhand-grip lat pulldown, 210, **210**
Uric-acid crystals, 24
Urination
  calcium loss through, 69–70
  hydration and, 73
Urine, 73

V

Vastus intermedius, 195, **195**
Vastus lateralis, 195, **195**
Vastus medialis, 195, **195**
Vegetables, 10, 91
Vegetarian diet
  compliance with, 102
  muscle loss from, 76
  testosterone decrease from, 76, 86
Vitamin B_6 supplementation, 177
Vitamins, fat-soluble, 12
VO_2 max, 35, 36

W

Warmup, 172–73, 178–79
  need for, 172–73
  raising core temperature with, 173
  strength-training, 41
  techniques for, 178
  workout, 199, 227, 256
Water loss, 69
Water weight, 66
Weight bench, 170, **170**
Weight gain, 98
Weight lifting
  avoiding bounce during, 199
  effects of
    cortisol decrease, 164
    flexibility increase, 180
    injuries, 168
    metabolic increase, 40
    muscle damage, 74
    testosterone increase, 40, 161
  intensity of, 30
  popularity of, 32, 39
  stretching and, 180–81
  warmup sets, 178–79

Weight loss
  causes of
    exercise, 155–56
    low-carbohydrate diets, 101–2
    low-fat diets, 102
  energy balance and, 100–101
  macronutrient balance and, 101
  mulitplier effect in, 104
Weight plates, **171**, 171–72
Welterweight
  grocery list, 144
  menus, 145–51
  protein shake, 115
Wide-grip lat pulldown, 270, **270**
Workout(s). *See also* Testosterone
    Advantage workout
  break from, 286
  duration of, 165
  eating before and after, 165
  finding new, 288
  frequency of, 165
  goal setting for, 287–88
  location considerations, 167–69
  periodized training, <u>292</u>

plateaus in, 285–86, 293
recovery from, 165
total-body vs. training split,
    290
variations, in
  exercises, 289
  intensity, 290–91
  order of exercises, 289–90
  training splits, 290
  volume, 290
  way of doing exercises, 289
Workout log
  phase 1, 199, **200–203**
  phase 2
    workout A, **230–31**
    workout B, **246–47**
  phase 3
    workout A, **260–61**
    workout B, **268–69**
    workout C, **276–77**

Z

Zinc supplementation, <u>177</u>
ZMA supplement, <u>177</u>